IMMUNOLOGY COLORING BOOK

Learn and enjoy coloring the components of the immune system.

INTRODUCTION

Your Immune system is the first line of defense against germs and it's the one that is keeping you alive. It's the main topic that help you understand the way your body defends itself and which way is better than learning it by coloring the different components of this magnificent system to get the general idea of it all.

This coloring book helps you to memorise the most of immunology cells and systems especially visual learners.

Immunology coloring book is well organized, starting from the principal components of the immune system (antibodies, LT and LB cells, macrophages, Dendritic cells, complement system components…) passing by the defense mechanisms of the body against germs and bacteria (activation of LB and LT cells, ADCC, Phagocytosis, Diapedesis…) arriving to the major immune system disorders (hypersensibility, HIV…) so you can dig deep and get the general idea of every cell's role and each immune response mechanism by coloring them.

This book offers the user the chance to learn and have fun.

TABLE OF CONTENT

I.   Cells of the immune system................... 5

II.   Primary Lymphoid organs 8
   1.Bone marrow
   2.Thymus

III.   Secondary Lymphoid organs................ 12
   1.Spleen
   2.Lymph node

III.   Cells of specific immunity................... 17
   -LT and LB cells activation mechanisms

IV.   Cells of innate immunity.................... 39
   -Monocytes and APC work mechanisms
   -Basophil ,Mast and Eosinophil cells

V.   Antigens..................................... 61

VI.   Complement system 63

VII. Major Histocompatibility Complex 66

VIII.Cell Adhesion Complex 69

IX.   Non self cell rejection 71

X.   Immunoglobulin 73

XI.   Hypersensibility 77

XII. Precipitation And Agglutination Reactions. 79

XIII.Monoclonal Gammopathie 81
   - Multiple Myeloma
   - Lymphoma CLL

XIV.Acquired Immunodeficiency Syndrome..... 86

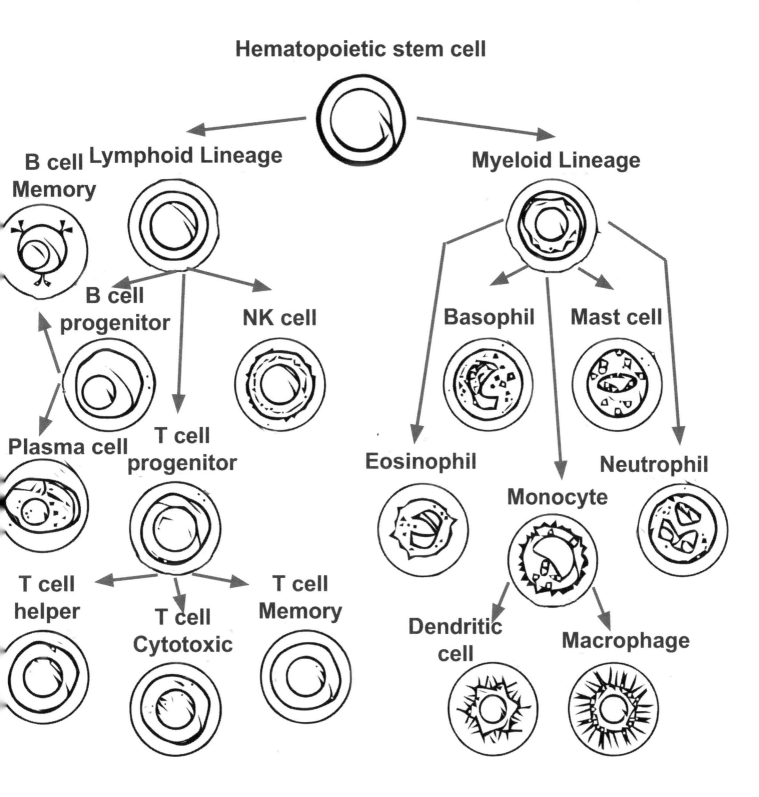

Cells of the Immune system   5

Innate (Non specific)
Fast response 0-4 hours

Mononuclear phagocyte system

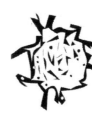

Macrophage

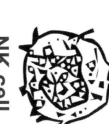

Dendritic cell

Monocyte

Complement protein

Granulocytes

Eosinophil   Neutrophil

Basophil

Mast cell

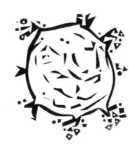

NK cell

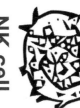

NK T cell

γδ T cell

Adaptive (Specific)
Late response 3-14 days

7

Humoral

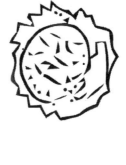

B cell

Antibody

Cellular

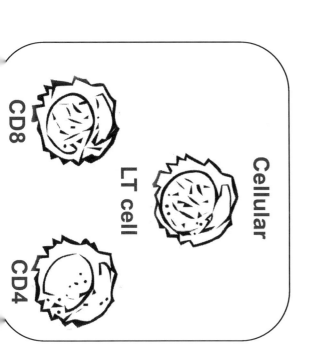

CD8

LT cell

CD4

Primary lymphoid organs

1. BONE MARROW:

It's the it origin of hematopoiesis and more specifically in the red marrow region.

LB cells are synthesized and maturated there, while LT cells continue their maturation in the thymus.

The myeloid lineage is specialized in the non specific immunity, and the lymphoid lineage is known for its specific immune response.

The two lineage work together for well being of the body.

Bone Marrow

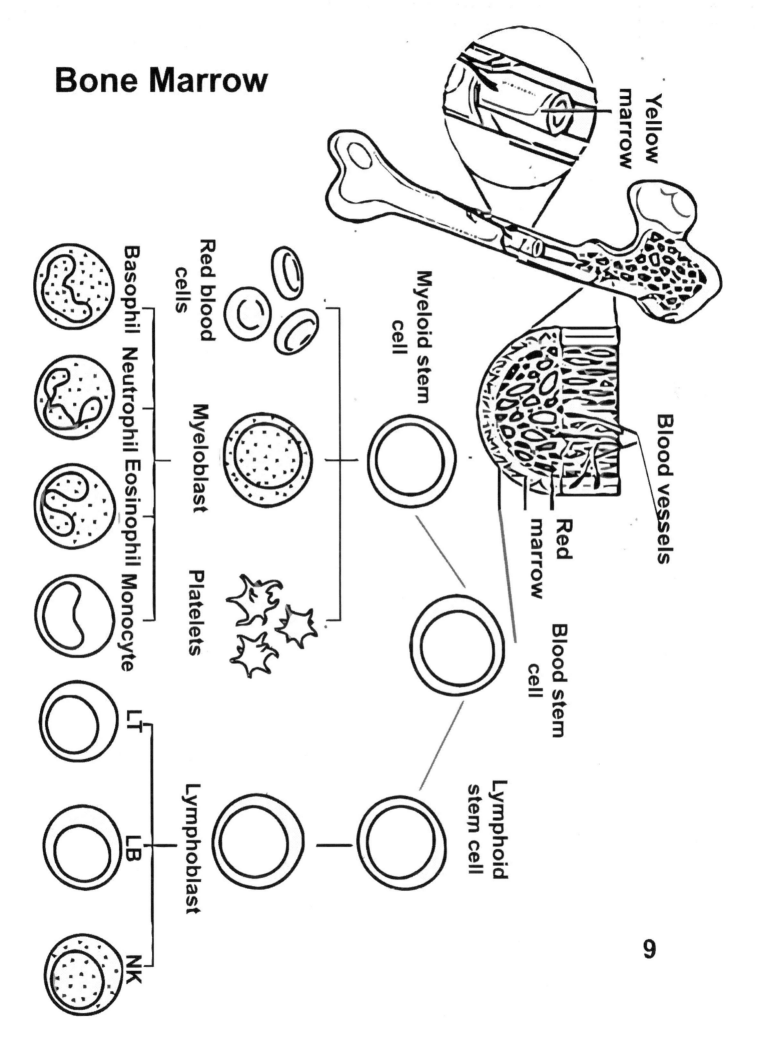

Yellow marrow

Blood vessels

Red marrow

Blood stem cell

Myeloid stem cell

Red blood cells

Myeloblast

Platelets

Basophil Neutrophil Eosinophil Monocyte

Lymphoid stem cell

Lymphoblast

LT

LB

NK

9

Primary lymphoid organs

2. THYMUS:

It's the site of LT cells differentiation and maturation, where it go throw a series of selections to define the cells that eligible to finish its maturation and those are the ones which recognise the MCH-peptide linkage.
It's formed of a cortex where immature LT cells are founded, and a medulla, the zone of mature LT.

Thymus

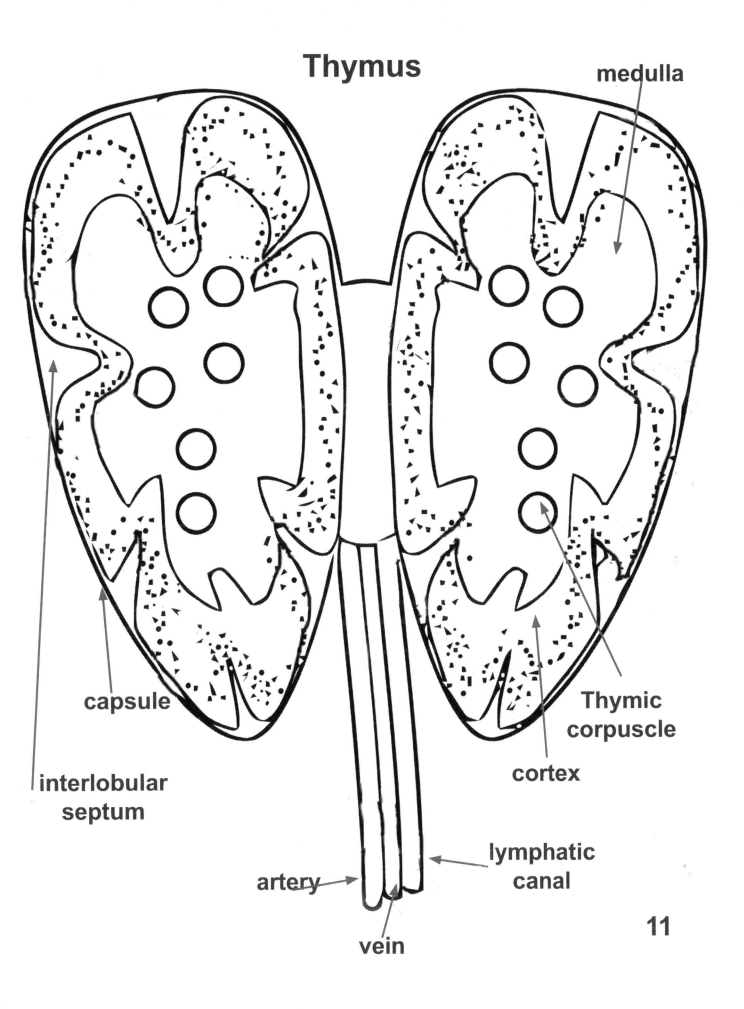

medulla

capsule

interlobular
septum

Thymic
corpuscle

cortex

artery

lymphatic
canal

vein

11

Secondary lymphoid organs

1. SPLEEN:

It's formed of the red pulp which is the the cemetery of the erythrocytes and the white pulp where LB and LT zone is founded.

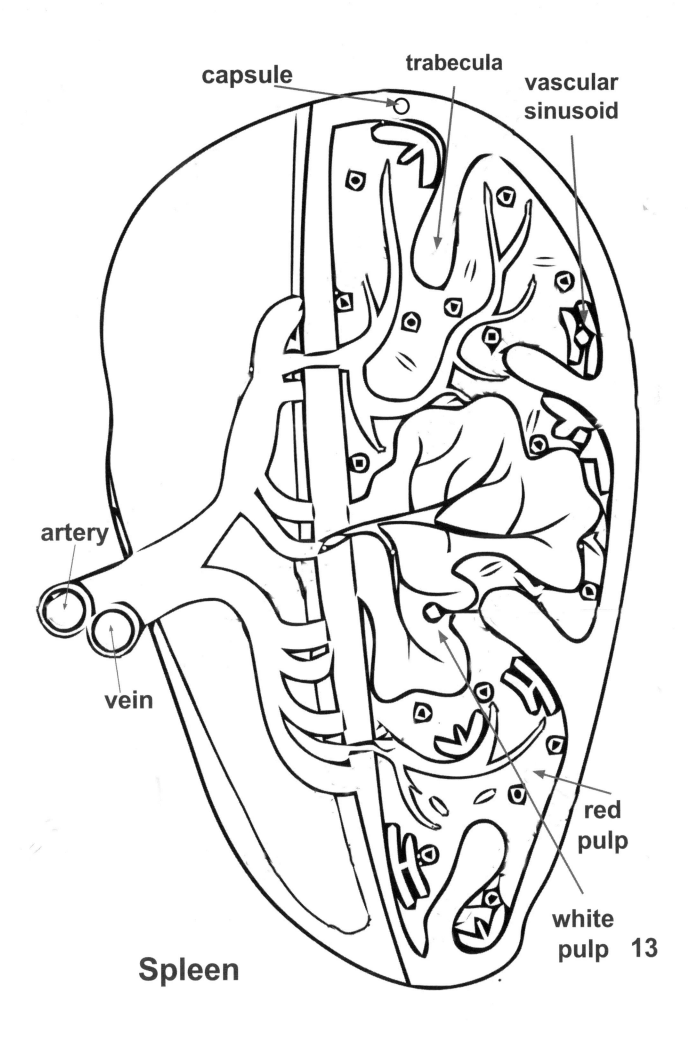

capsule

trabecula

vascular
sinusoid

artery

vein

red
pulp

white
pulp   13

Spleen

Secondary lymphoid organs

2. LYMPH NODE:

It's the place where antigen and immune cells meet up.
It's formed of a cortex where LB cells are found in crowns to form primary follicles and transforms into secondary follicles after Ag stimulation, a Para-cortex which is rich in LT cells, and a medulla where the humorale T-dependant response takes place.

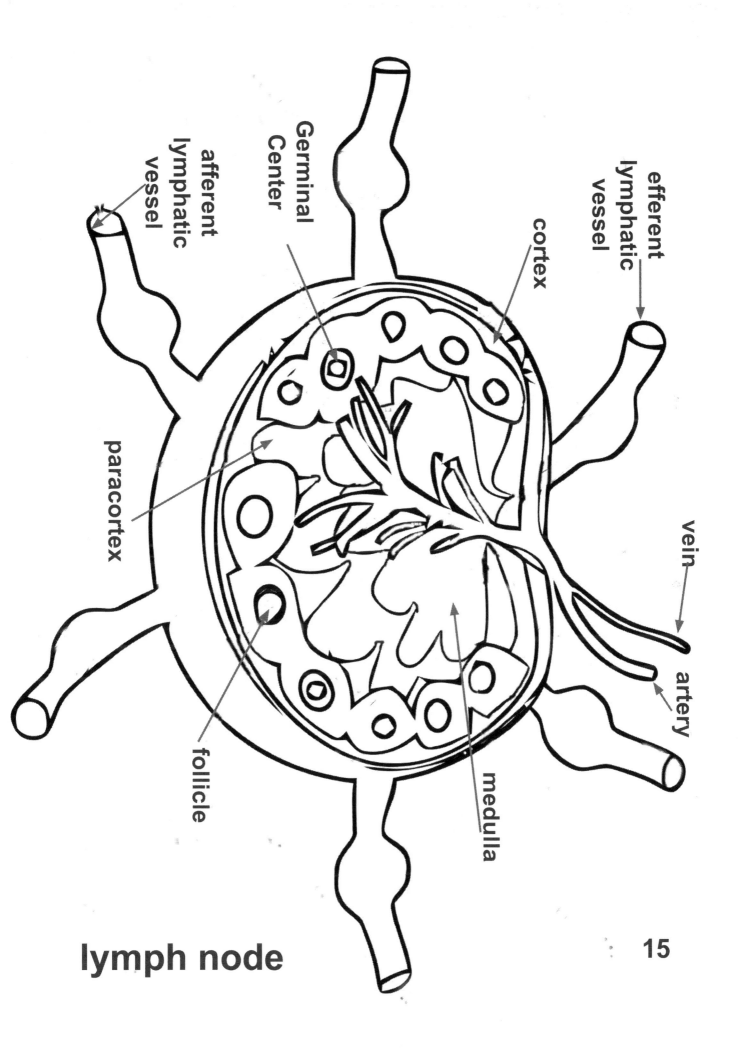

afferent
lymphatic
vessel

Germinal
Center

efferent
lymphatic
vessel

cortex

paracortex

vein

artery

follicle

medulla

lymph node

15

CELLS OF SPECIFIC IMMUNITY

1. LT cells:

LT cells are specialized in cellular adaptive immunity, there is mainly a naive T cell that produces LTCD4 which is a T helper cell, activating cellular and humoral immunity thanks to the cytokines that it releases; and the LTCD8 which kills the infected and cancer cells after being activated by LTCD4.

LT CELLS TYPES

Native LT
Newly produced with no contact with an Antigen

Regulation LT
Prevents autoimmune diseases

Memory LT
Produced after first contact with the Antigen

LT Helper
Help LTs to mature

CD4

LT cytotoxic
kill infected and tumor cells

CD8

17

CELLS OF SPECIFIC IMMUNITY

Activation of LT cells:

When a microbe gets into the body, it gets phagocytosed by APC cells and presented to LTCD4 cell by recognition of TCR receptor and MHC II on one hand, and CD28 with CD80-CD86 on the other hand. The LTCD4 will synthesize cytokines which will activate LTCD8 and help it replicate and kill the infected cell.
Memory LT cells will be formed at the same time.

Activation of LT cells

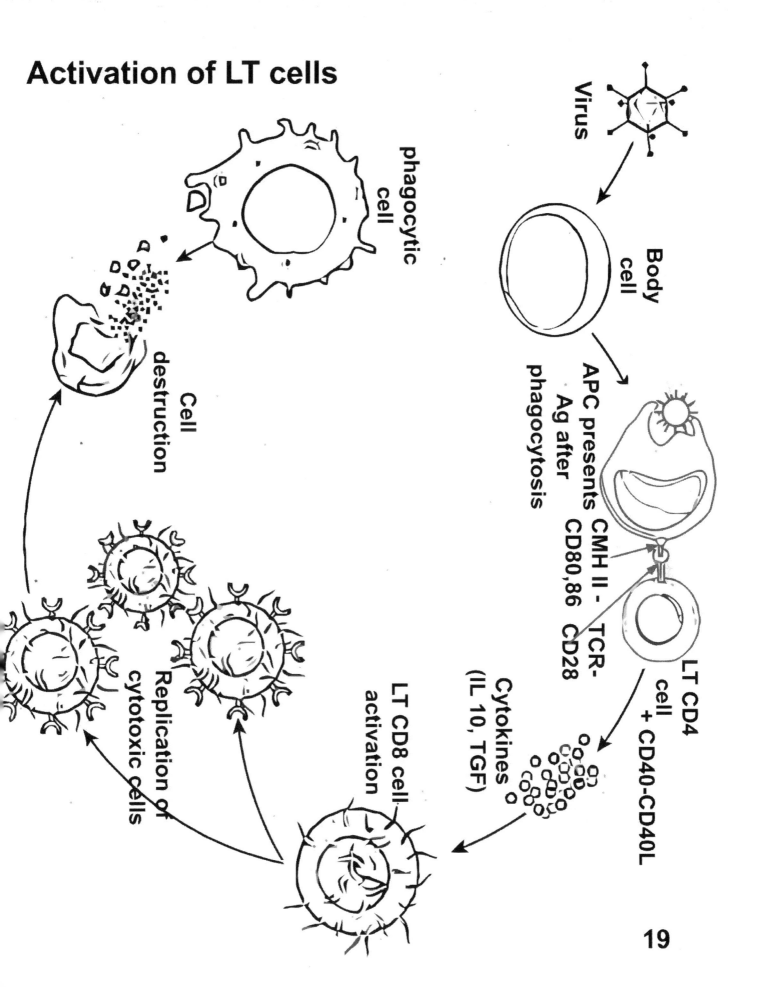

Virus

Body cell

phagocytic cell

APC presents Ag after phagocytosis

CMH II - TCR-
CD80,86   CD28

LT CD4 cell
+ CD40-CD40L

Cytokines
(IL 10, TGF)

LT CD8 cell activation

Replication of cytotoxic cells

Cell destruction

19

CELLS OF SPECIFIC IMMUNITY

Actions of LTCD8 cells:

When LTCD8 recognize the infected cell throw the complex TCR-MHC I / Peptide-CD8 , it will start its lytic mechanisms by releasing perforins and granzymes which will destroy the cell by creating apoptotic bodies.

Actions of LT CD8

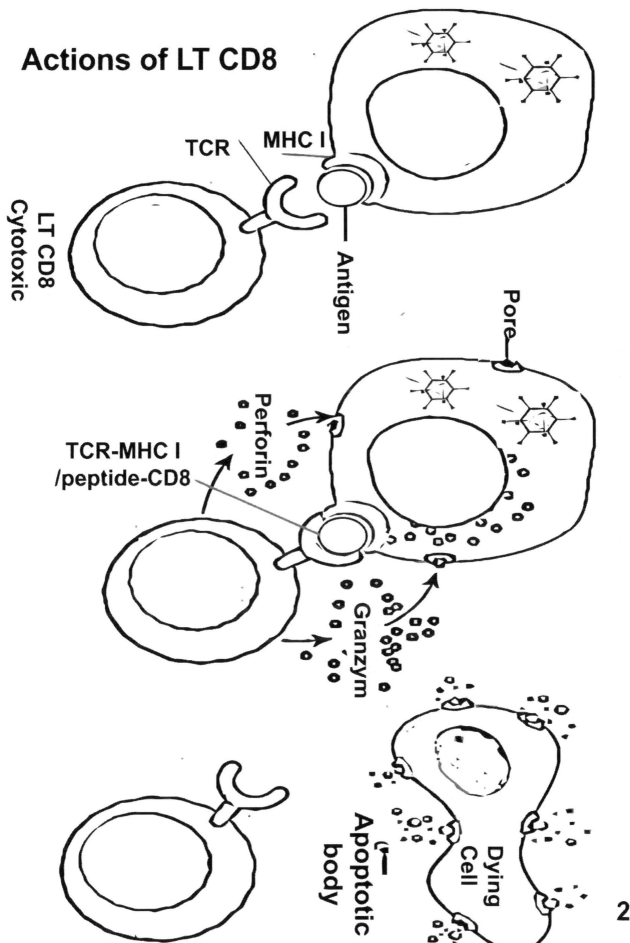

21

CELLS OF SPECIFIC IMMUNITY

LTCD4 Helper:

After the phagocytation of the microbe and presenting its antigen to the LTCD4 cell (TH0), the TH0 will differentiate into a TH1 cell and TH2 cell.
TH1 is the progenitor of the cellular immunity by releasing IL2, IL12, TNF β and IFN γ which will activate the cytotoxic cells.
TH2 will activate the humoral immunity by synthetizing IL 4 5 6 10 13 which will help transforming B cells into plasma cells and releasing Ig.

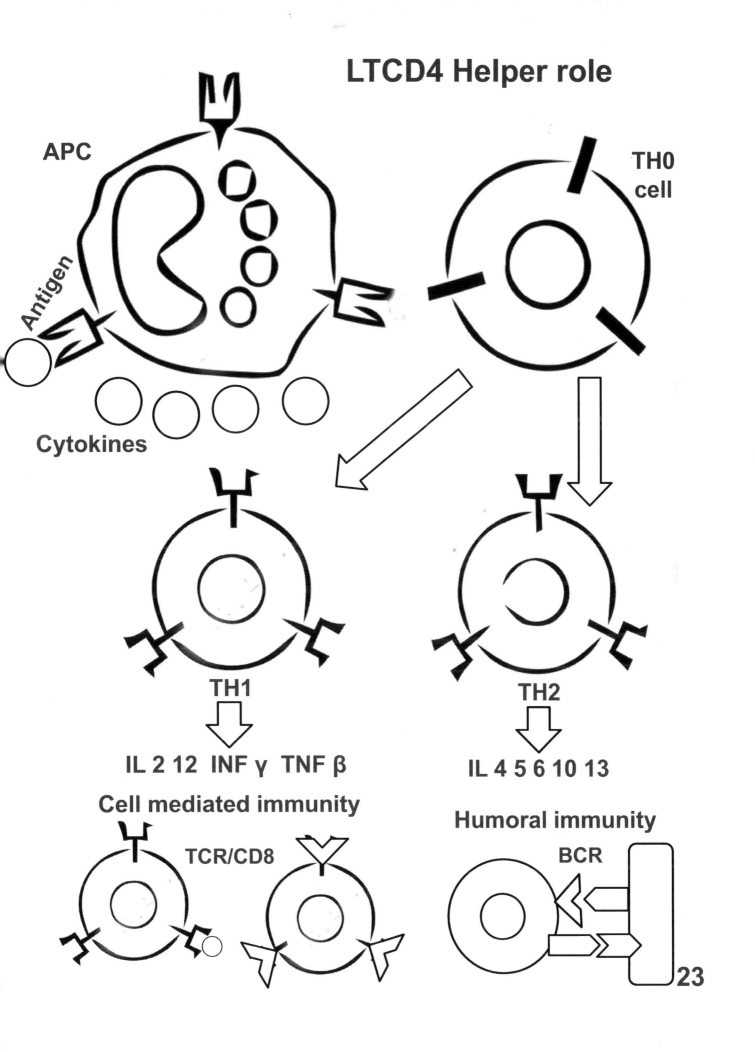

CELLS OF SPECIFIC IMMUNITY

Natural Killer cell:

A Natural cytotoxicity cell: anti-viral and anti-tumor, with no specificity to an antigen, and no specific receptor to it.
It contains cytotoxic intracytoplasmic granules: Perforin and granzymes which will destroy the targeted cell.
It secrets IFNy and TNF alpha.

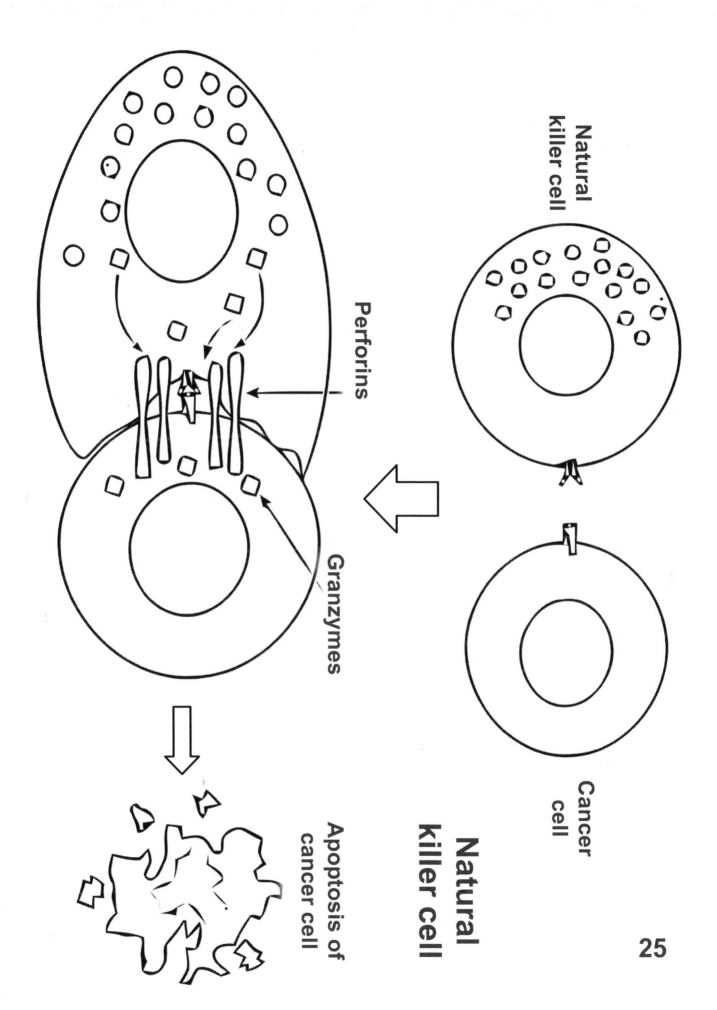

Natural
killer cell

Cancer
cell

Natural
killer cell

Perforins

Granzymes

Apoptosis of
cancer cell

25

CELLS OF ADAPTIVE IMMUNITY

ADCC:

The antibody dependant cellular cytotoxicity is specialized in elimination cancer cells and infected cells. It starts by binding of the antybody to the antigen, then a NK cell recognise and bind to the functional region of the antibody, the NK cell will start releasing the perforins and granzymes to destroy the cancer cell by apoptosis.

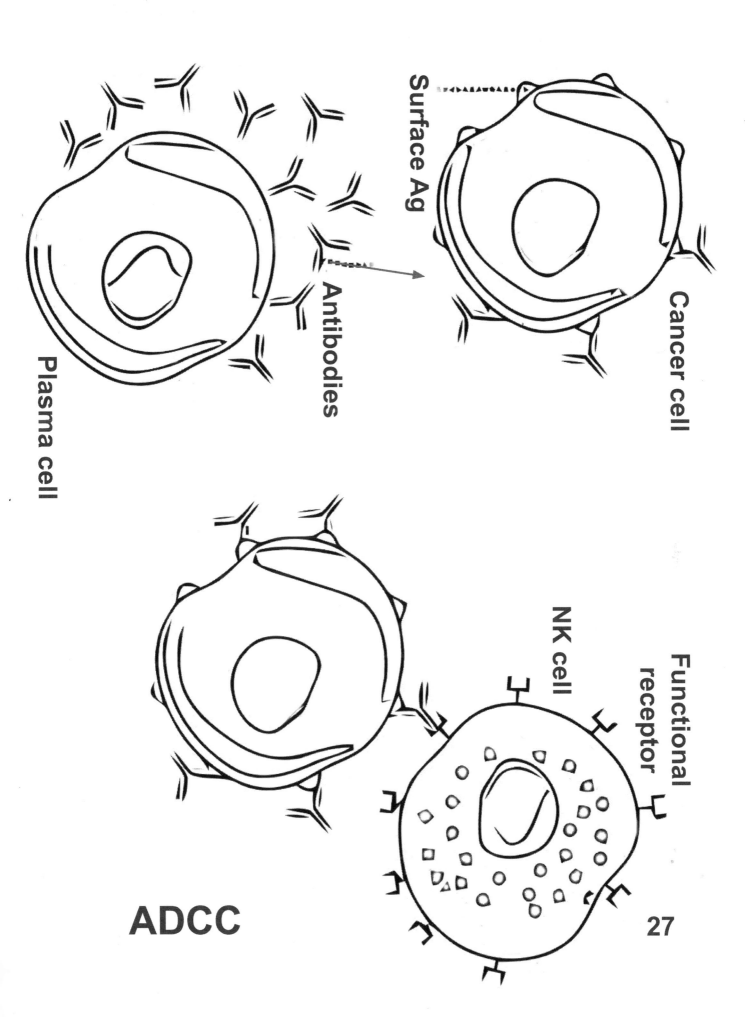

Plasma cell

Antibodies

Surface Ag

Cancer cell

NK cell

Functional receptor

ADCC

27

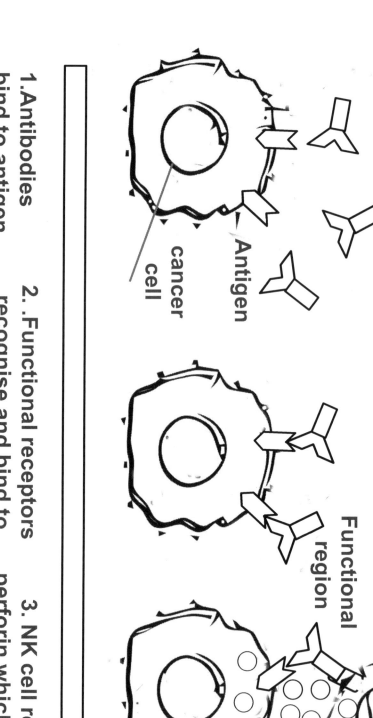
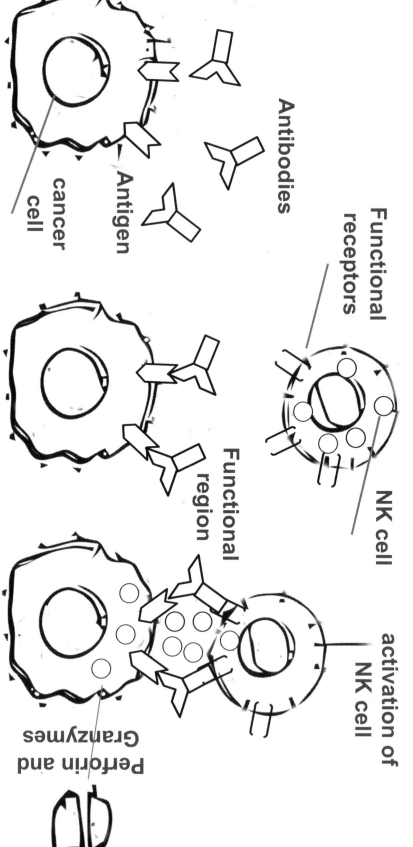

1.Antibodies bind to antigen

2..Functional receptors recognise and bind to the reciprocal portion of an antibody

3. NK cell release perforin which causes the lysis of the cancer cell

4..Apoptosis of cancer cell

Antibodies

cancer cell

Antigen

Functional receptors

NK cell

Functional region

activation of NK cell

Perforin and Granzymes

ADCC 28

CELLS OF SPECIFIC IMMUNITY

LB cell:

LB cells are specialized in humoral adaptive immunity. LB is the origin of plasma cells which will produce Ig cells, and Memory LB cells to respond immediately in case of a second infection by the same Ag.

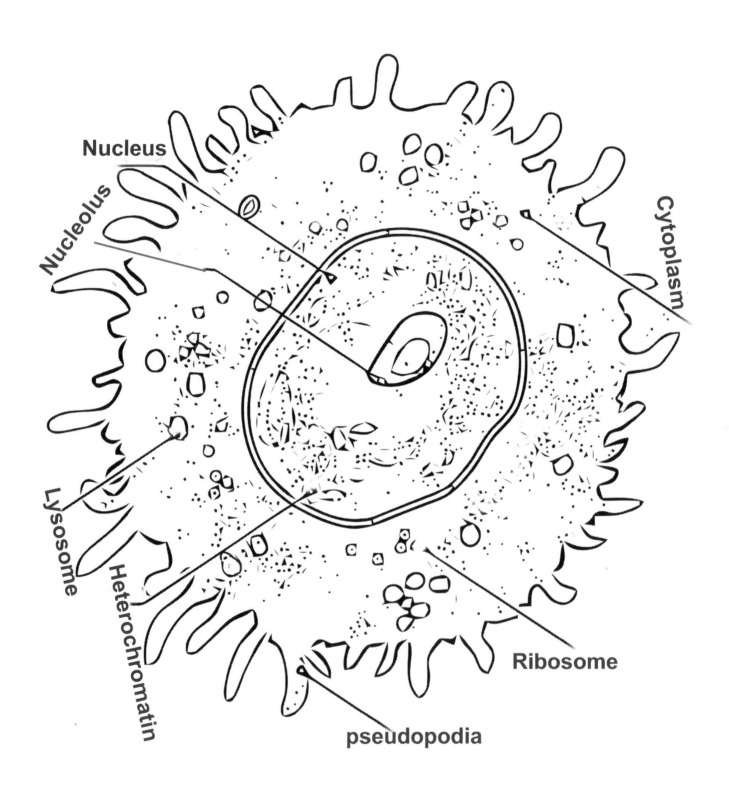

Nucleus

Nucleolus

Cytoplasm

Lysosome

Heterochromatin

Ribosome

pseudopodia

Naive LB cell

30

CELLS OF SPECIFIC IMMUNITY

Plasma cell:

It's the source of immunoglobulins which is the main actors of the humoral immunity, it's produced after activation LB cell by cytokines.

Plasma cell

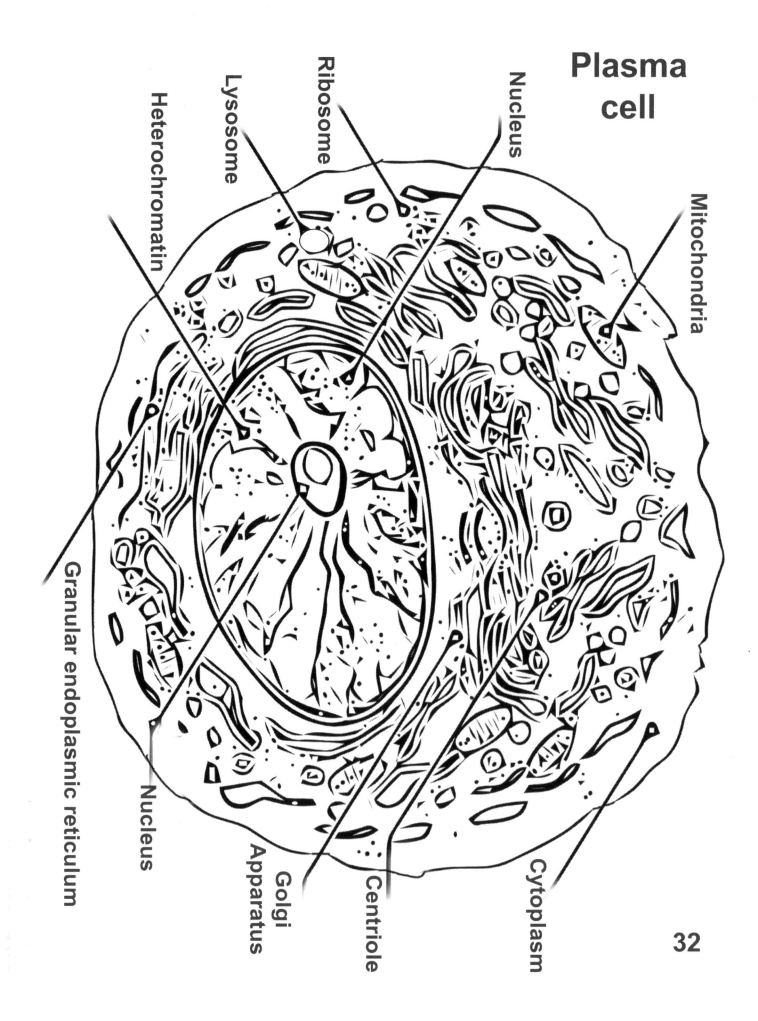

Ribosome

Lysosome

Heterochromatin

Nucleus

Mitochondria

Granular endoplasmic reticulum

Nucleus

Golgi Apparatus

Centriole

Cytoplasm

CELLS OF SPECIFIC IMMUNITY

Thymo-independent activation of LBs :

This type of activation does not require TH2 to produce antibodies (IgM) and does not induce memory:
- Polyclonal proliferation of LBs (activation of receptors common to all LBs except BCR) by mitogenic Ag
- Monoclonal proliferation of LBs (BCR activation) by repetitive sugar determinants.

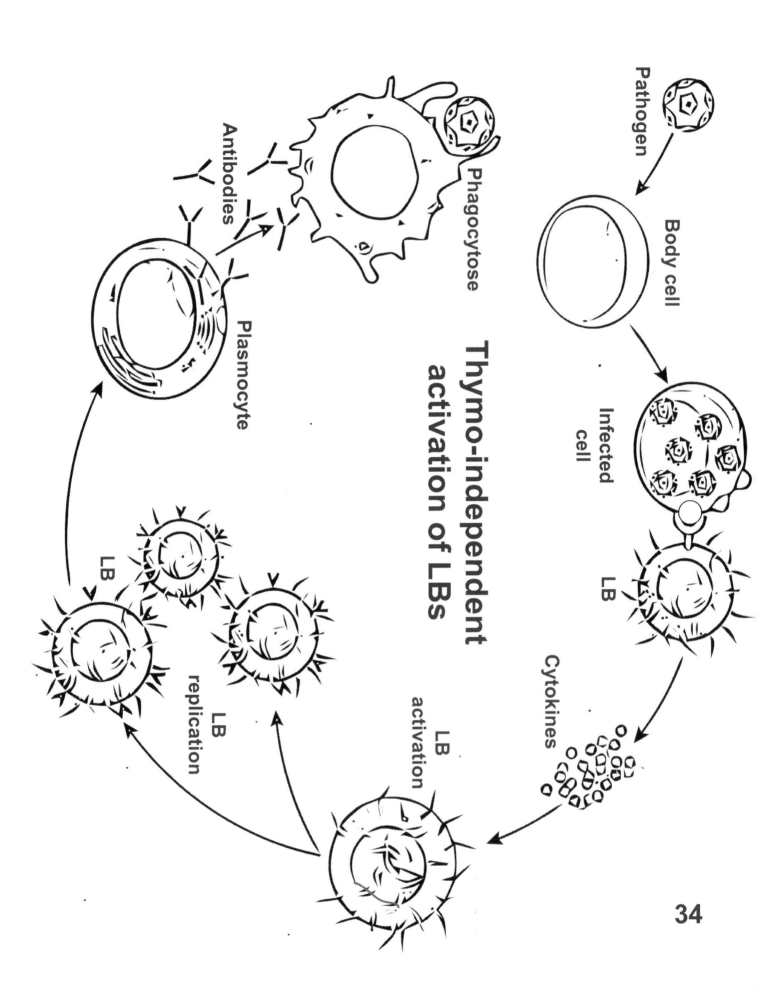

Thymo-independent activation of LBs

Pathogen

Body cell

Infected cell

LB

Cytokines

LB activation

LB replication

LB

Plasmocyte

Antibodies

Phagocytose

34

CELLS OF SPECIFIC IMMUNITY

Thymo-dependent activation of LBs (majority of responses):

After phagocytisis of the virus by APC, it will excrete IL1 to activate LT helper
- Specific recognition of the Ag by the BCR and its internalization
- LT-LB cooperation:
  Primary signal:
MHC-peptide-TCR interaction
  Costimulatory signal:
B7-CD28 and CD40-CD40L (CD154)
  Cytokine production: IL-4, IL-5 to activate LBs

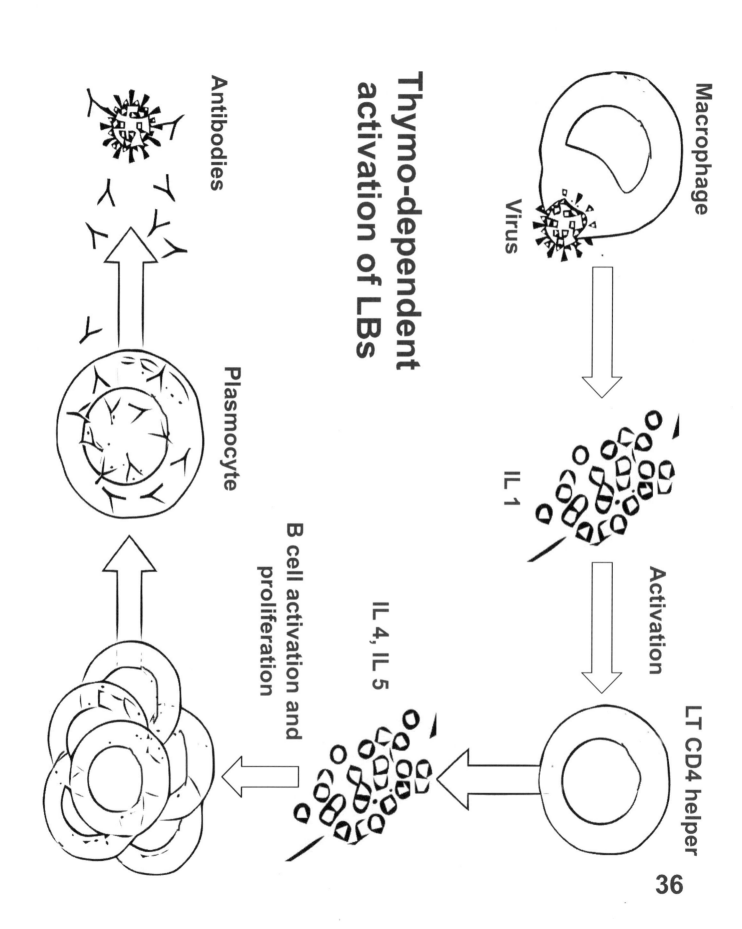

Thymo-dependent activation of LBs

Macrophage

Virus

IL 1

Activation

LT CD4 helper

IL 4, IL 5

B cell activation and proliferation

Plasmocyte

Antibodies

36

CELLS OF SPECIFIC IMMUNITY

Adaptive and innate immunity work together in a harmony to destroy virus and microbes starting by phagocytizing the virus by an APC to present an antigen to LTCD4 cell and help activate both cellular and humoral immunity.

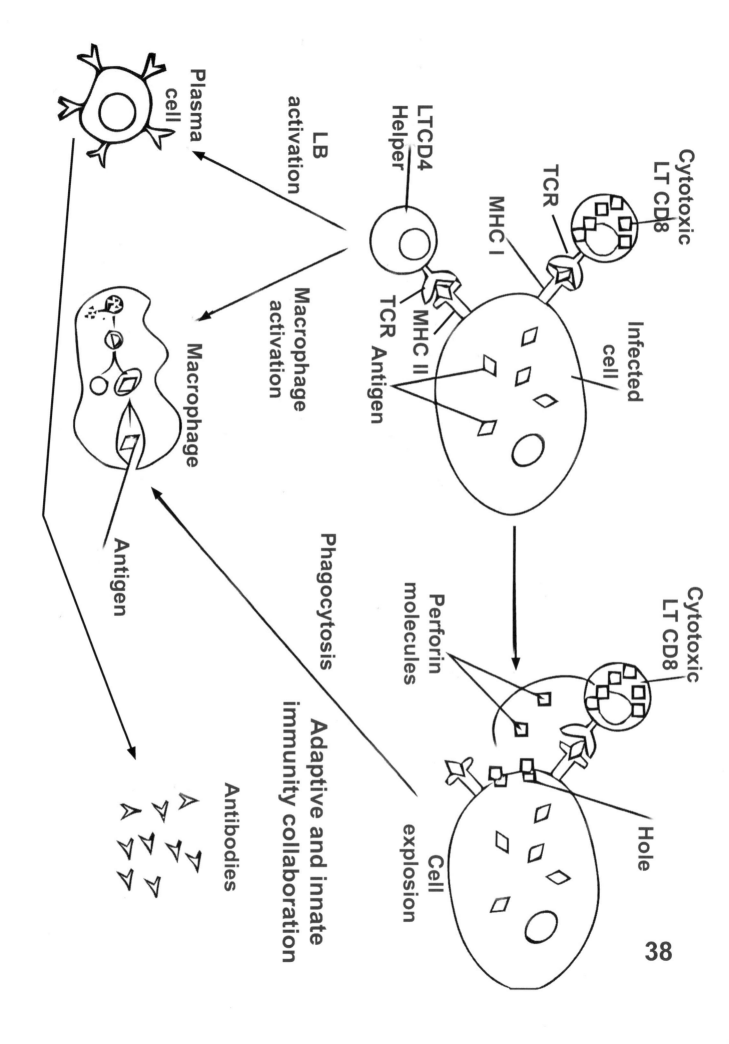

Plasma cell

LB activation

LTCD4 Helper

Cytotoxic LT CD8

TCR

MHC I

MHC II

TCR Antigen

Macrophage activation

Infected cell

Macrophage

Phagocytosis

Antigen

Perforin molecules

Adaptive and innate immunity collaboration

Antibodies

Cell explosion

Cytotoxic LT CD8

Hole

38

CELLS OF INNATE IMMUNITY

Monocytes:

Monocytes are the main source of the antigen presentatrice cells, they represented by macrophages in the tissues, Kupffer cells in the liver, histiocytes in the connective tissue, synovial cells in the synovial capsule, microglial cells in nervous tissue, alveolar cells in the lungs, Osteoclast in the Bone, Mesangial cells in the Kidney.

MONOCYTE

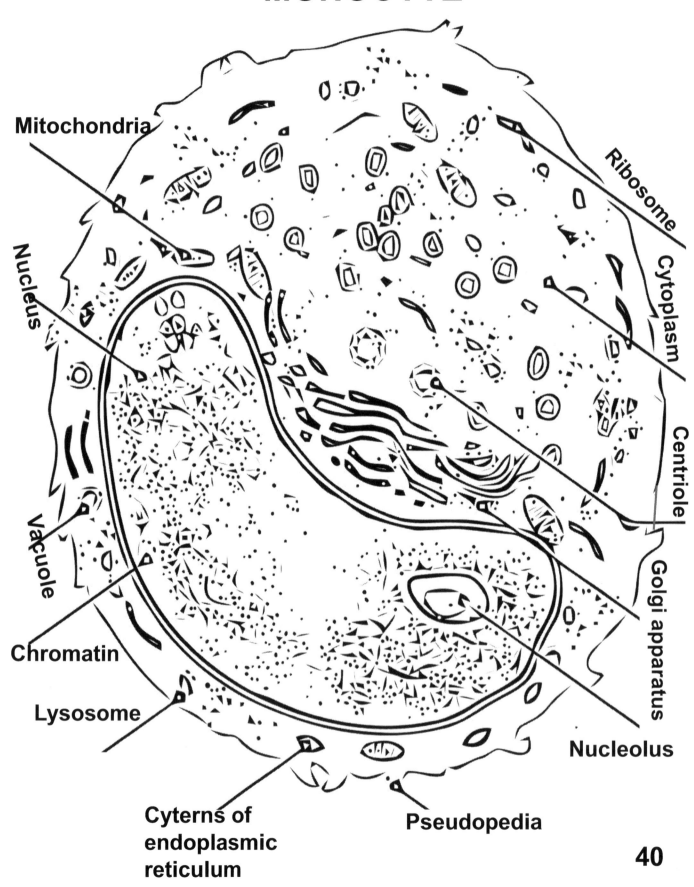

Mitochondria

Ribosome

Nucleus

Cytoplasm

Centriole

Golgi apparatus

Vacuole

Chromatin

Lysosome

Nucleolus

Cyterns of
endoplasmic
reticulum

Pseudopedia

40

CELLS OF INNATE IMMUNITY

Monocytes:

Monocytes differentiate and produce macrophages, dendritic cells, osteoclast, Kupffer cells, histiocytes, synovial cells, microglial cells, alveolar cells.
It's the most important cell of the myeloid lineage.

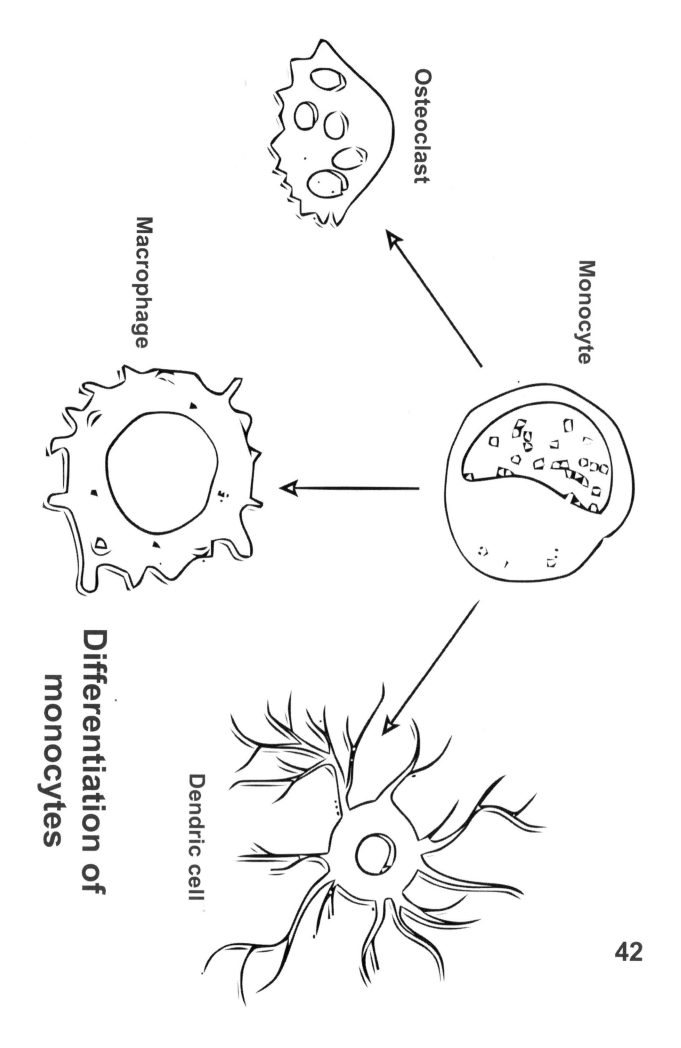

Osteoclast

Monocyte

Macrophage

Dendric cell

Differentiation of monocytes

42

CELLS OF INNATE IMMUNITY

Monocytes:

Monocytes are the origin of macrophages throw two essential ways:
- Macrophages classically activated by LPS and INF γ
- Macrophages alternatively activated by IL4 and IL14 .

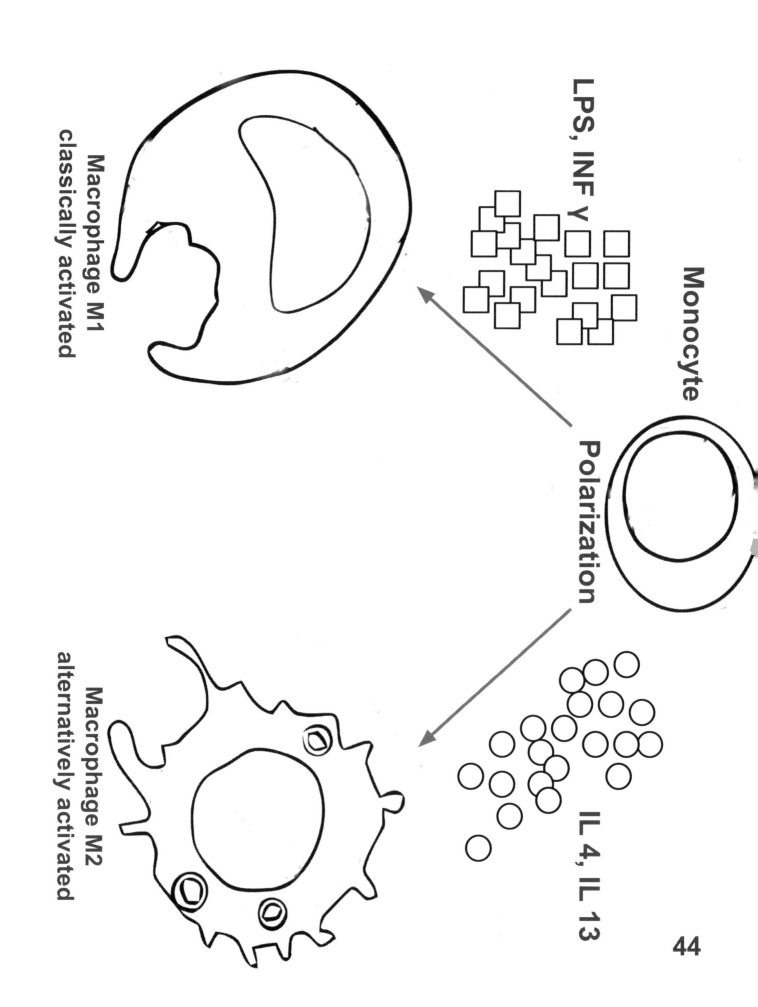

Monocyte

Polarization

LPS, INF γ

Macrophage M1
classically activated

IL 4, IL 13

Macrophage M2
alternatively activated

44

CELLS OF INNATE IMMUNITY

Macrophages:

Derives from blood monocytes, responsable for multiple tasks: presentation of Ag to LT cell, phagocytosis, Antibody dependent cellular cytotoxicity. The presentation of Ag is about
- Peptides from Ag degradation are presented to LTs by MHC molecules
- IFNy activates macrophages: Increases expression of HLA I and II molecules, and potentiates cytokine production by macrophages.

Macrophage

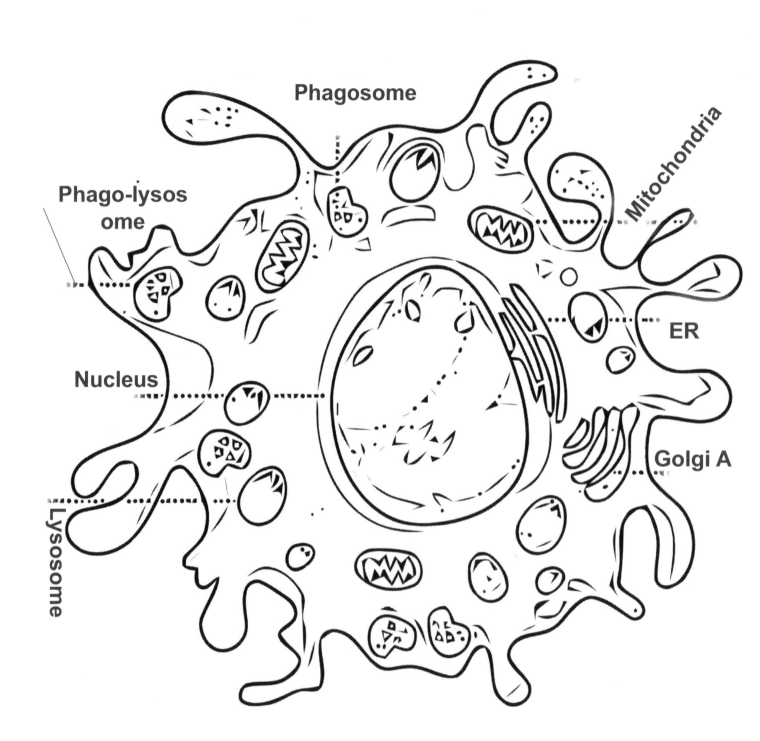

Phagosome

Mitochondria

Phago-lysos
ome

Nucleus

ER

Lysosome

Golgi A

CELLS OF INNATE IMMUNITY

Phagocytosis :

It's a process through which APC activate LTs to start eliminating microbes .
It starts by forming pseudopods - phogosome - phagolysosome - microorganism destroyed by enzymes - cellular debris released by exocytosis.

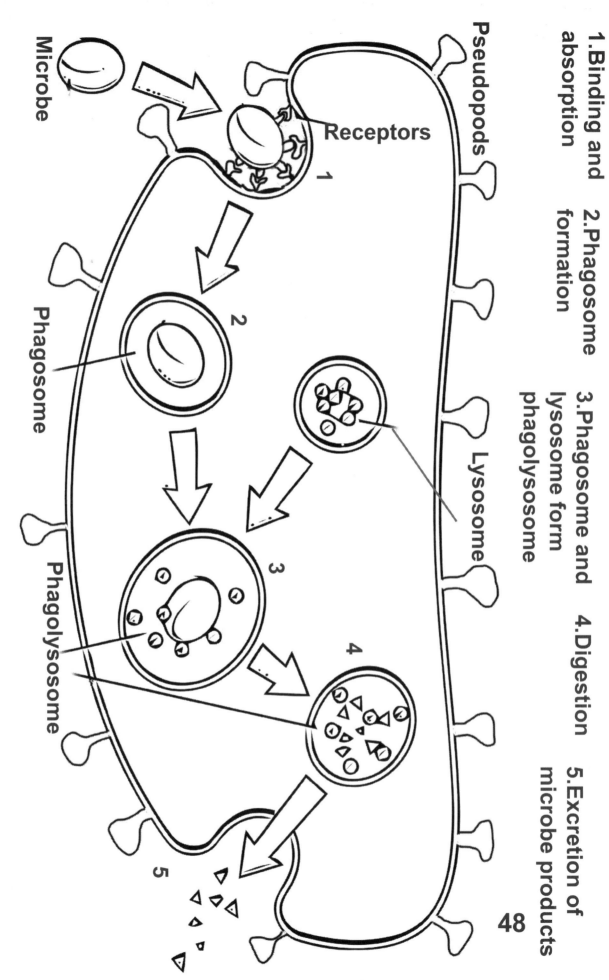

Phagocytosis

1.Binding and absorption

2.Phagosome formation

3.Phagosome and lysosome form phagolysosome

4.Digestion

5.Excretion of microbe products

Pseudopods

Receptors

Microbe

Phagosome

Lysosome

Phagolysosome

48

CELLS OF INNATE IMMUNITY

Neutrophil cells :

Represents the vast majority of leukocytes in the blood.
It is the first phagocytic cell to mobilize to eliminate microbes.
It is a Bactericide of extracellular bacteria, it's responsable of clearance of immune complexes.

Neutrophil cell

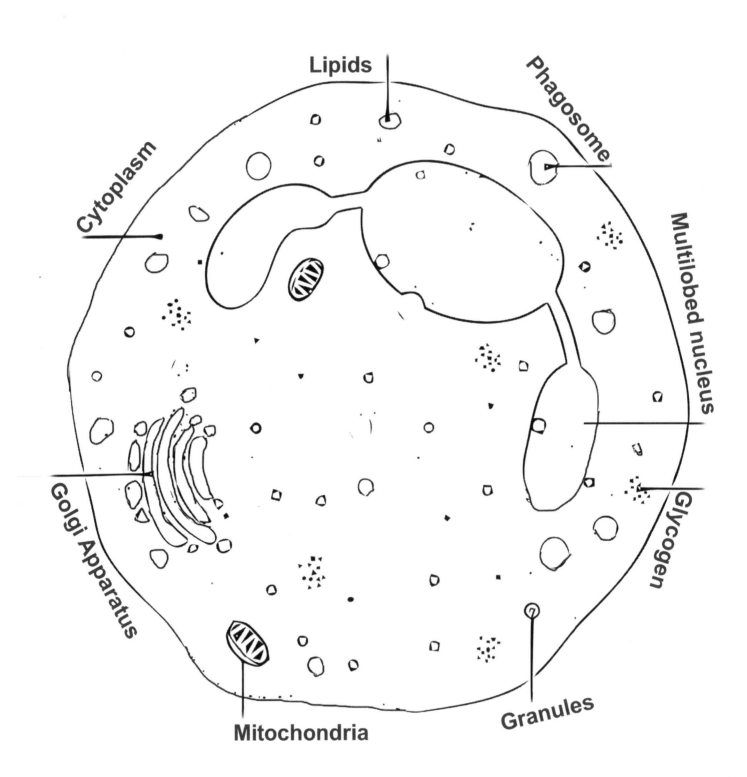

Lipids

Phagosome

Cytoplasm

Multilobed nucleus

Golgi Apparatus

Glycogen

Mitochondria

Granules

50

CELLS OF INNATE IMMUNITY

Diapedesis :

It's the passage of leukocytes between two endothelial cells from the blood vessel to get to the infection site.
It's preceded by adhesion, tight binding and follow-up by migration to the infection site where it excrets cytokines, phagocyte the microbe and degranulate its contents.

Diapedesis

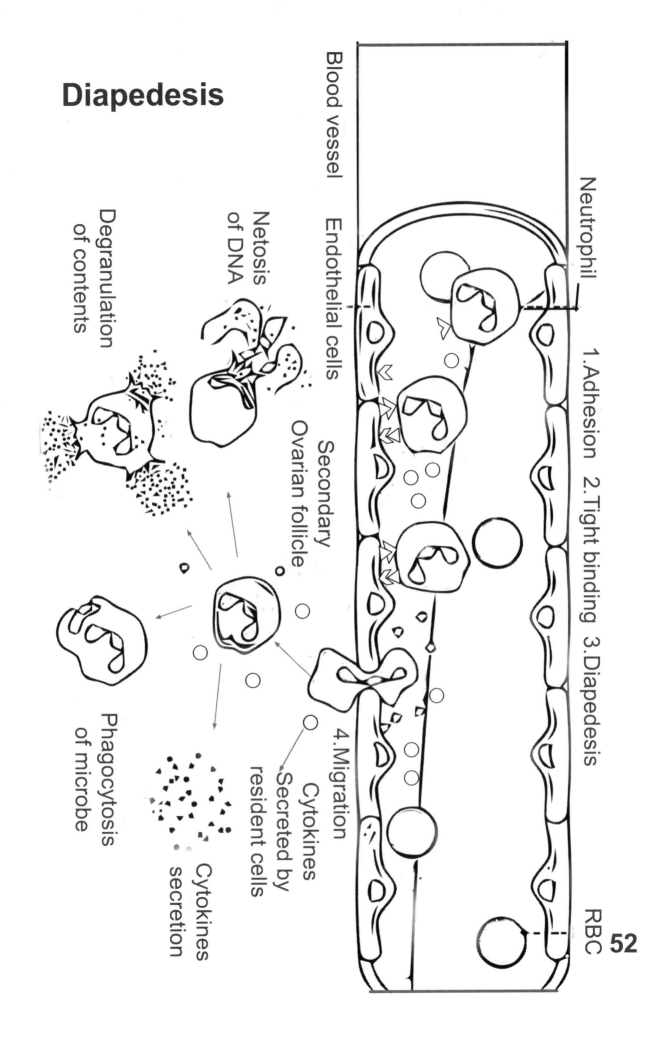

Blood vessel

Endothelial cells

Netosis
of DNA

Degranulation
of contents

Secondary
Ovarian follicle

Phagocytosis
of microbe

Cytokines
secretion

4.Migration

Cytokines
Secreted by
resident cells

Neutrophil

1.Adhesion 2.Tight binding 3.Diapedesis

RBC 52

CELLS OF INNATE IMMUNITY

Eosinophil cells:

It's a cytotoxic cell located mainly in tissues (skin, muq), with a brief passage in the blood.

Main agent in the fight against certain parasites.

Participates in anaphylactic reactions and it's increased in certain vasculitides.

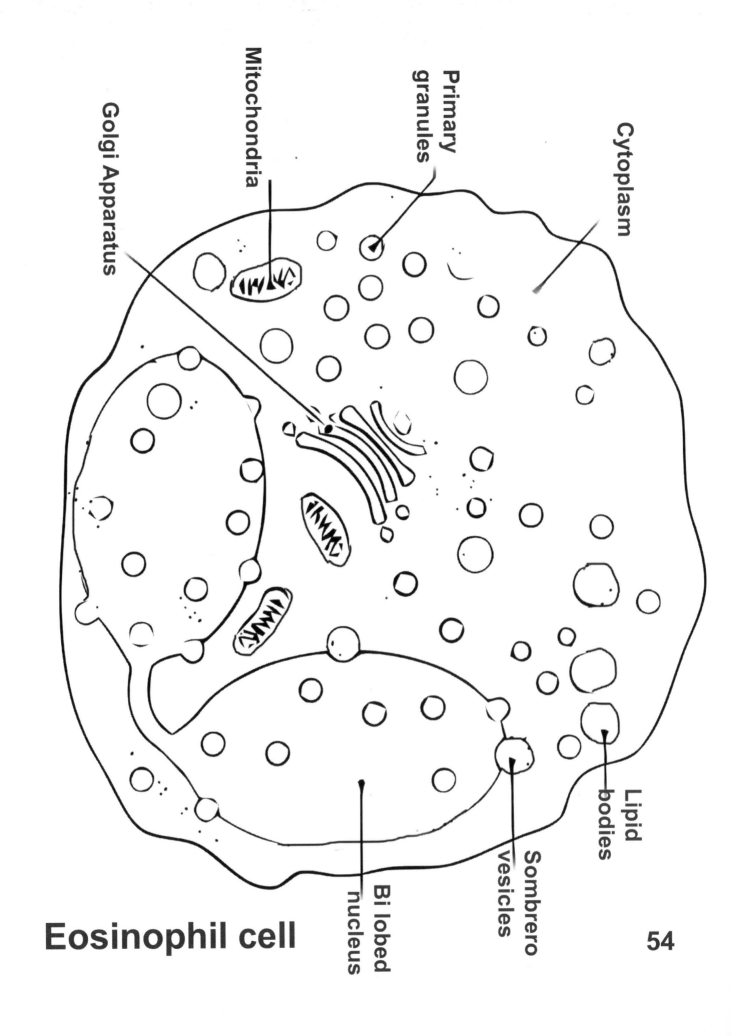

Mitochondria

Primary
granules

Cytoplasm

Golgi Apparatus

Bi lobed
nucleus

Sombrero
vesicles

Lipid
bodies

Eosinophil cell

54

CELLS OF INNATE IMMUNITY

Basophil cells:

These cells exit the bone marrow as mature cells, it Expresses receptors for IgE, with an important role in defense mechanisms against certain parasites. Participate in IgE dependent and IgE independent anaphylaxis reactions.

Basophil

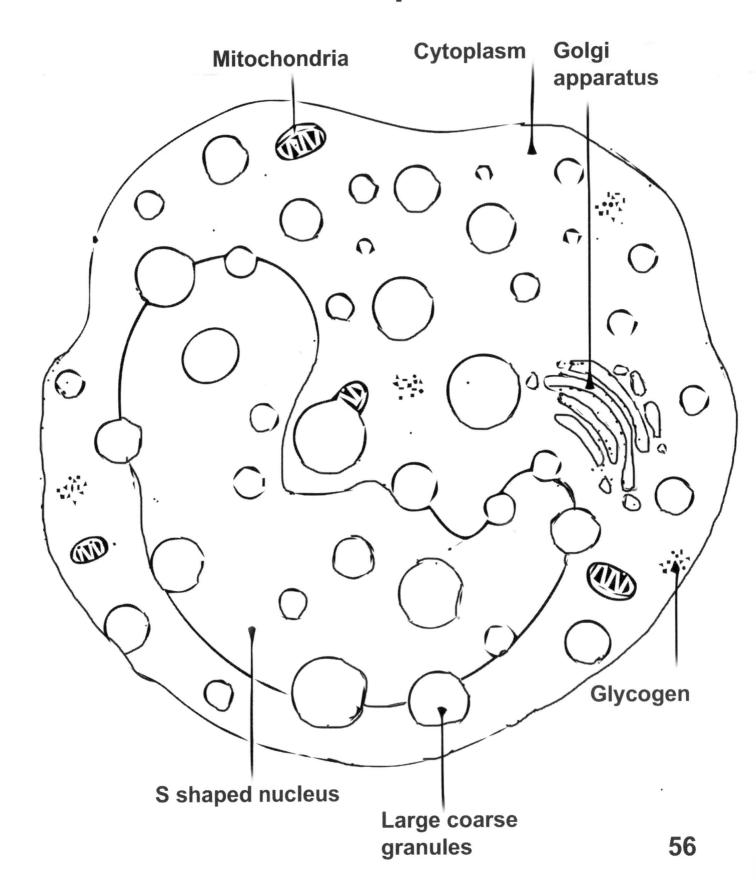

Mitochondria

Cytoplasm

Golgi apparatus

Glycogen

S shaped nucleus

Large coarse granules

56

CELLS OF INNATE IMMUNITY

Dendritic cells:

Professional Antigen Presenting Cells as they are the only ones able to stimulate naive LTs, and able to activate naive and memory LBs
it's found in the Blood as circulating DC, in the Epithelium as Langerhans cell, in the Lymphatic circulation (afferent channels) as veiled cells: T-zone of LOII, in Lymphoid organs (interdigitated cells), in Thymus : cortico- medullary junction, in the Spleen as periarteriolar sleeve of the white pulp, Lymph nodes paracortex + MALT in the subepithelial and interfollicular zone, lymphoid follicles : (follicular DC) capture immune complexes and present them to LBs.
DCs exist in 2 different states:
Immature DCs in tissues: no MHCII, role in endocytosis and antigen retrieval
Mature DCs in LOII T-zones: MHCII, presentation of MHC-Peptide complexes to LTs.

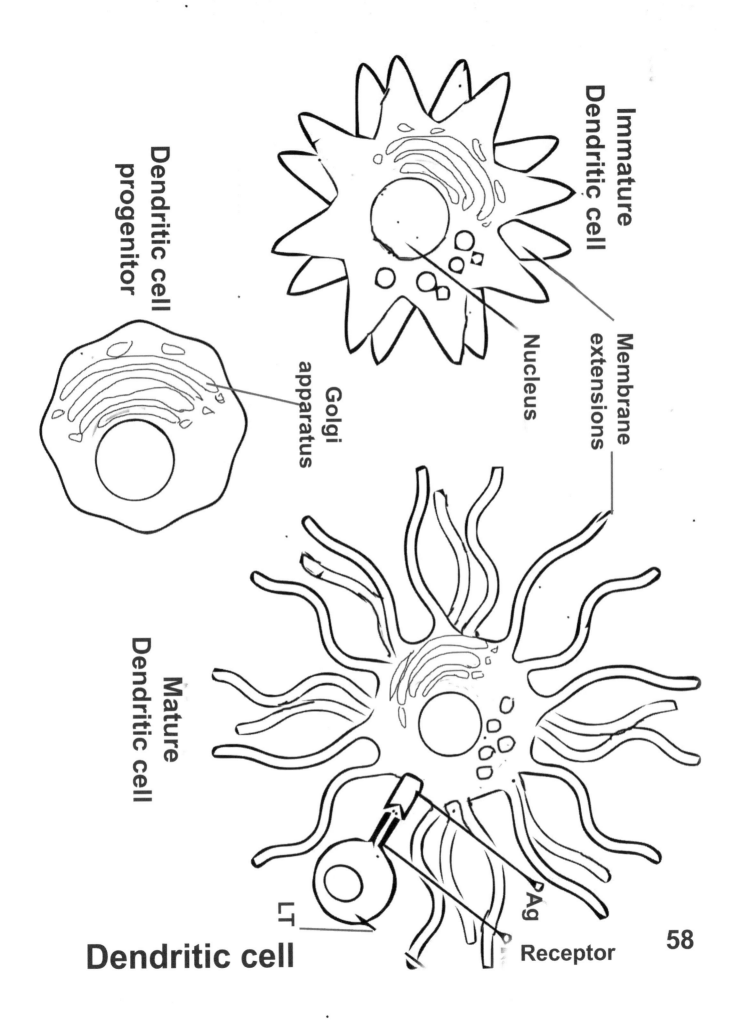

Immature
Dendritic cell

Dendritic cell
progenitor

Golgi
apparatus

Nucleus

Membrane
extensions

Mature
Dendritic cell

LT

Ag

Receptor

Dendritic cell

58

CELLS OF INNATE IMMUNITY

Mast cell:

It has a Large cytoplasmic granulations, it passes Briefly in the blood, it's found mainly in tissues.
It has a high affinity receptor for IgE and receptors for some complement degradation products.
It fights against certain parasites.

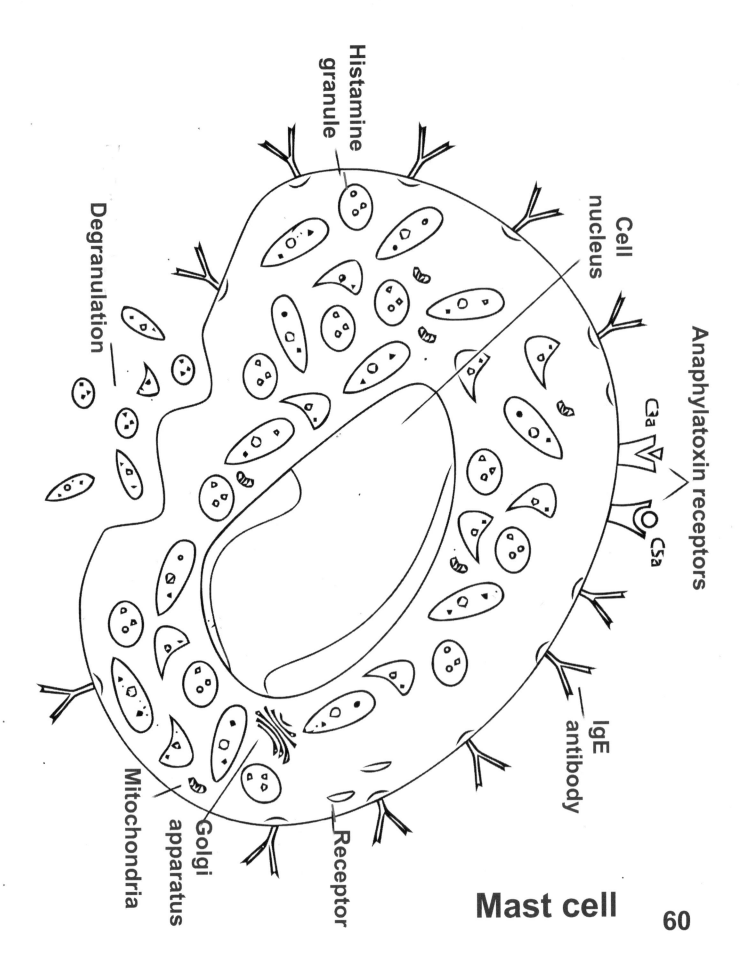

Histamine granule

Cell nucleus

Anaphylatoxin receptors

C3a

C5a

IgE antibody

Receptor

Golgi apparatus

Mitochondria

Degranulation

Mast cell

60

ANTIGENS

Induce an immune response: immunogenicity

Be recognized by an antibody or a lymphocyte (T or B): antigenicity

Immunization : induction of an immune response by inoculation of an immunogenic substance

Antigenic determinant = epitope: site responsible for antigenic reactivity. An antigen generally has several different epitopes. complementary structure with paratope (on Antibody)

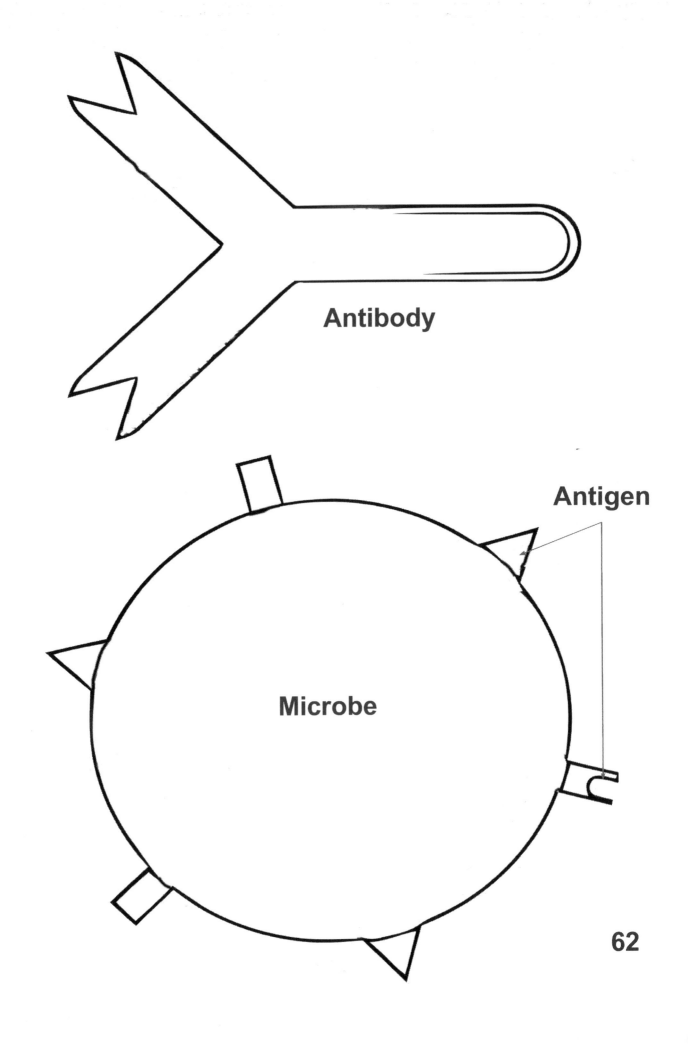

Antibody

Antigen

Microbe

62

COMPLEMENT SYSTEM

Plasma and membrane proteins, thermolabile, with opsonization-phagocytosis activity

The schema below explains how each pathway gets activated.

it's made of three pathways and each one has its own characteristics.

Complement system is made to do: Cell lysis, Opsonization -phagocytosis, Inflammation, Interface between innate and adaptive immunity: LB activation

V.COMPLEMENT SYSTEM

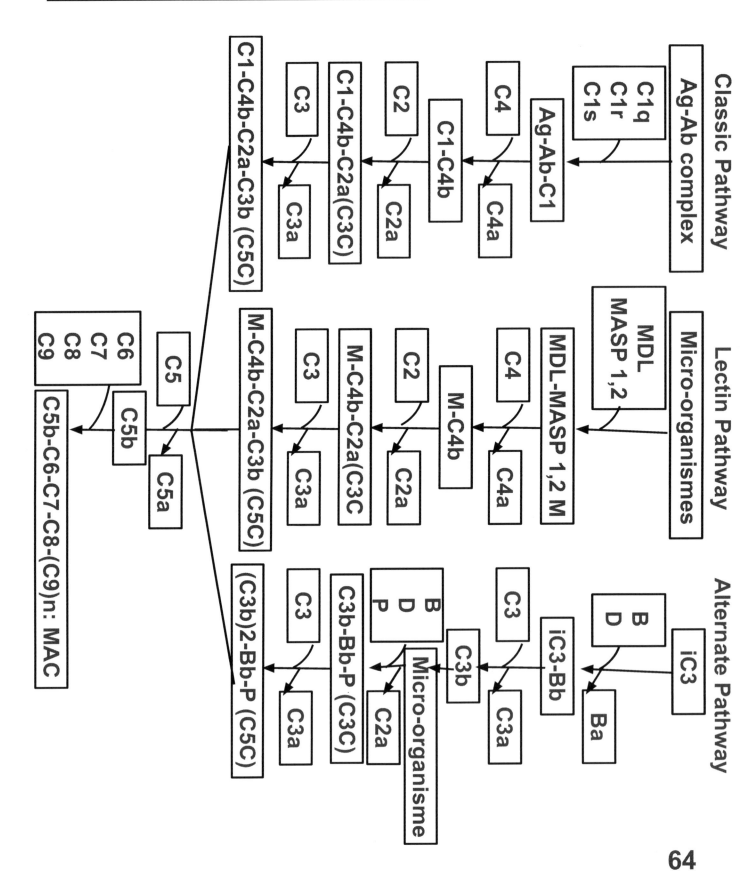

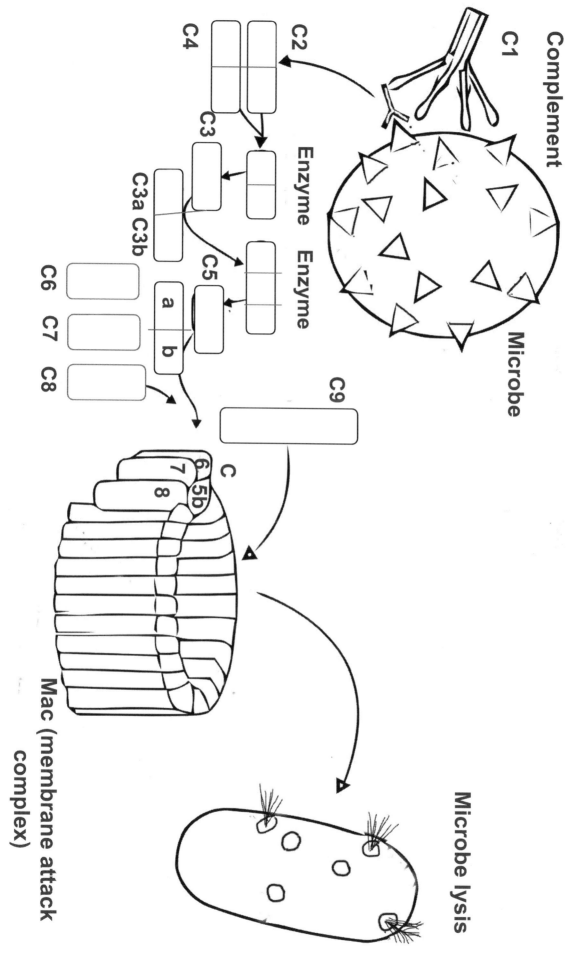

Complement

C1

C2

C4

C3

Enzyme   Enzyme

C3a C3b

C5

a

b

C6

C7

C8

C9

Microbe

Mac (membrane attack complex)

Microbe lysis

65

Major Histocompatibility Complex

Immunogenic and highly polymorphic membrane glycoproteins encoded by a series of genes
called MHC = HLA: multigenic, multi-allelic and codominant expression group.
Located on the short arm of chromosome 6.
HLA I: ubiquitous, most nucleated cells. > Absent : RBC, neurons, bone, cartilage.
HLA II: Restricted to certain cells
    APC: LB, monocytes/mac, dendritic cells (Langerhans, interdigital cells of the ganglion)
    LT after activation

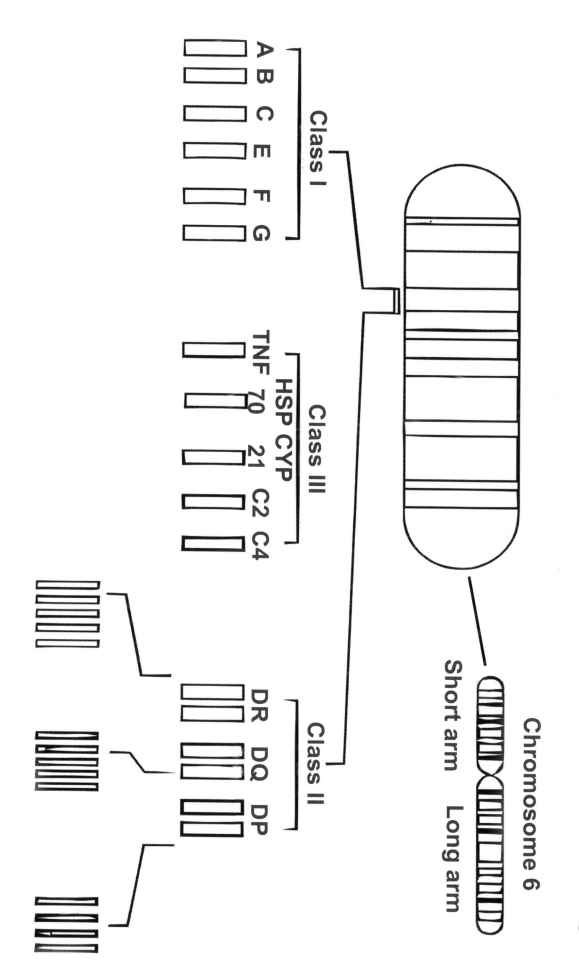

Class I

A
B
C
E
F
G

Class III

TNF
HSP 70
CYP 21
C2
C4

Class II

DR
DQ
DP

Chromosome 6

Short arm

Long arm

67

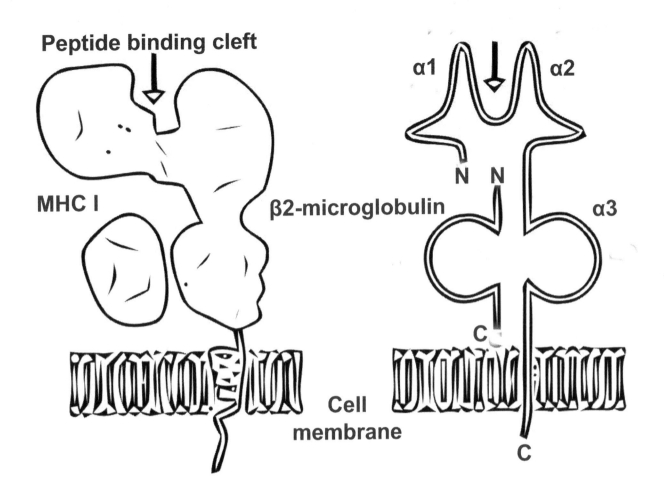

Peptide binding cleft

MHC I

β2-microglobulin

α1 α2

N N

α3

C

C

Cell membrane

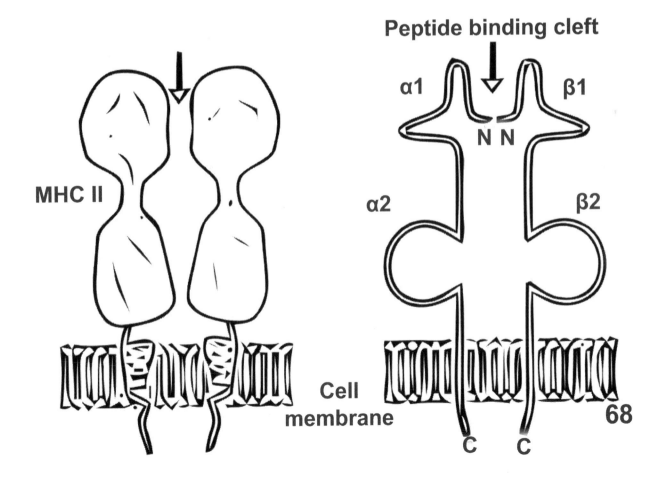

MHC II

Peptide binding cleft

α1 β1

N N

α2 β2

C C

Cell membrane

68

CELL ADHESION MOLECULES

Transmembrane glycoproteins (insoluble) expressed by leukocytes, endothelial C and platelets
5 main families : Selectins, integrins, mucins, cadherins and immunoglobulin superfamily

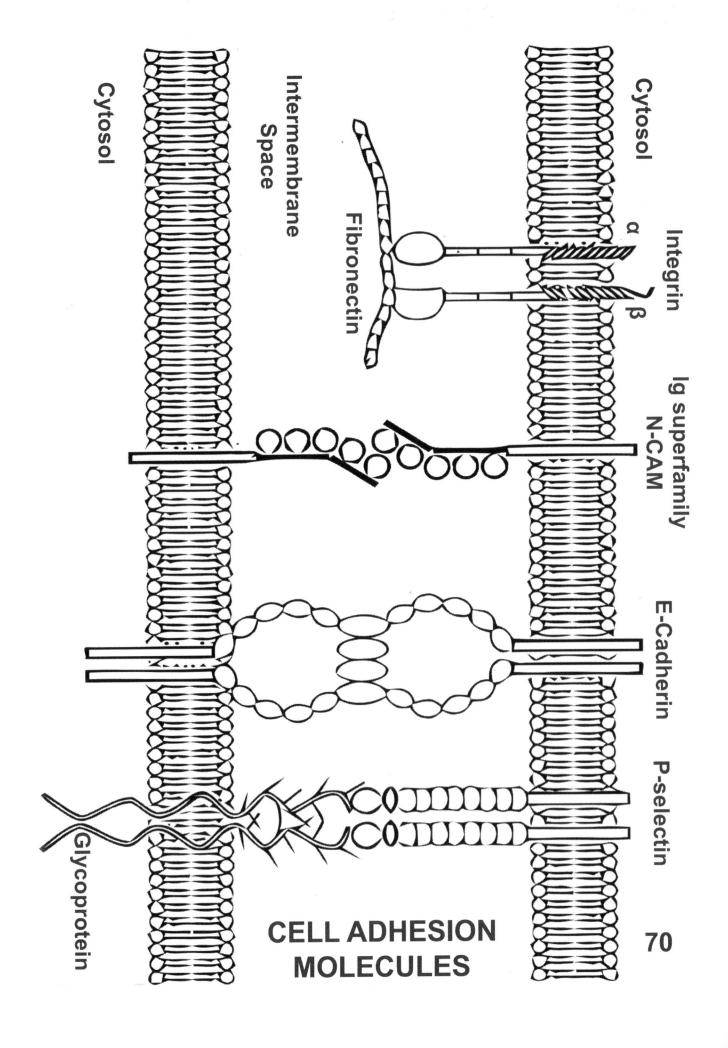

CELL ADHESION MOLECULES

70

Non self cell rejection

The rejection of a cell or an organ is defined by wether the cell has an inhibitory receptor on the cell to no get attacked by NK cells.

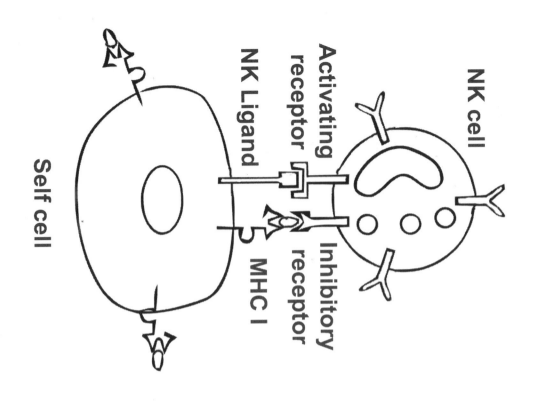

NK cell

Activating receptor

NK Ligand

Inhibitory receptor

MHC I

Self cell

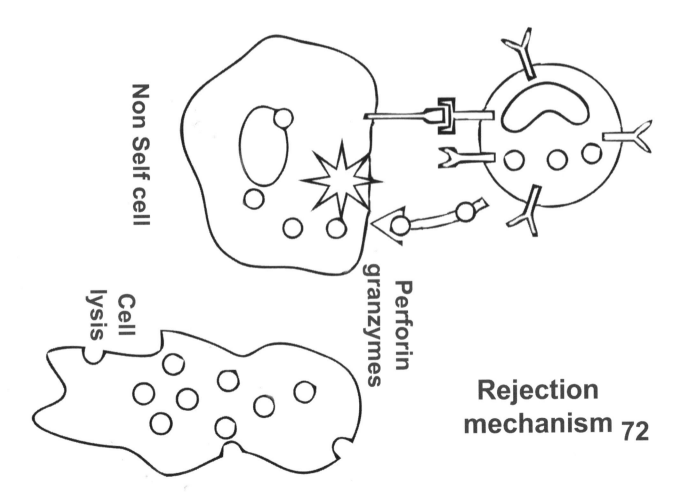

Non Self cell

Perforin granzymes

Cell lysis

Rejection mechanism 72

IMMUNOGLOBULIN

Globular glycoprotein produced by plasma cells
Exists in soluble form in biological fluids, and in membrane form: BCR
EPS: beta gamma zones
Extreme heterogeneity (homogeneity is pathological)
Genes coding for immunoglobulins: independent

- Kappa: Chromosome 2
- Lambda: Chromosome 22
- Heavy chains: Chromosome 14: VDJC: V (variable), C (constant), J (junction), D (diversity) genes. It has many functions;
    Recognition function: Carried by the Fab
- Active site (paratope): CDR (hypervariable Aa region) and FR (framework): Variable framework
- Size of the active site: 10 aa
- Antigen-antibody interaction is based on: complementarity and affinity
- Complementarity: no covalency, only Van Derwals, ionic, hydrophobic, hydrogen forces
- Cross-reactivity: an antibody recognizes 2 epitopes on several Antigens, or epitope of similar structure = Auto immune disease

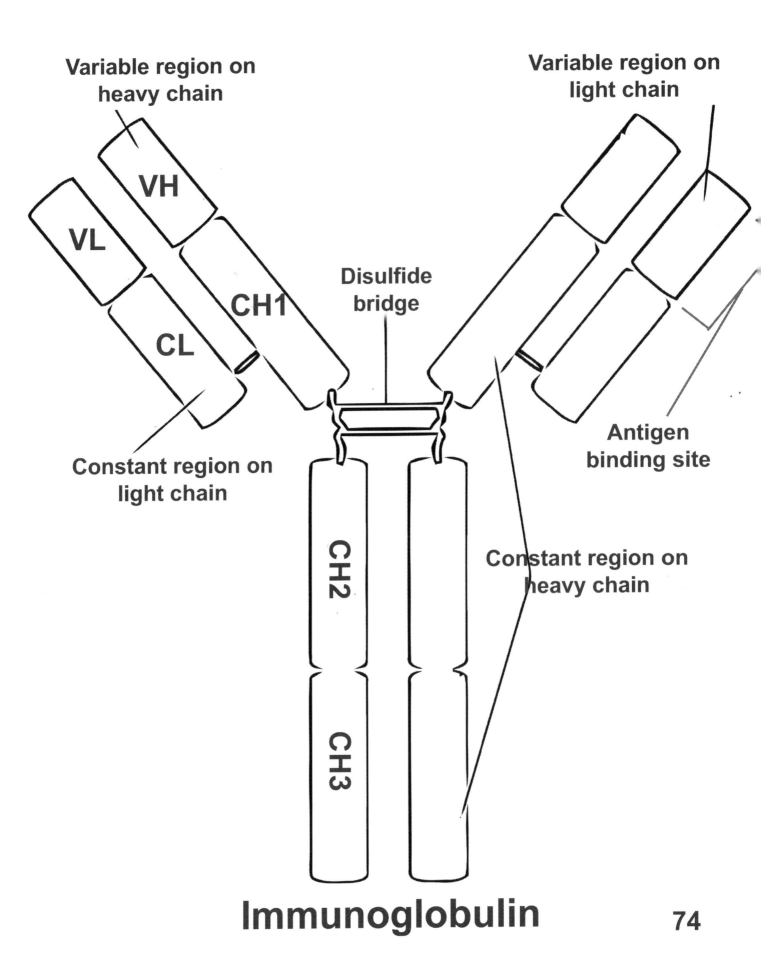

Variable region on heavy chain

VH

VL

CH1

CL

Disulfide bridge

Constant region on light chain

Variable region on light chain

Antigen binding site

CH2

CH3

Constant region on heavy chain

Immunoglobulin

74

IMMUNOGLOBULIN

1. IgG:
   - Subclasses: γ1,2,3,4
   - Alternate pathway: Aggregate: agglutinating
   - Cellular fixation: NP, Monocyte, Macrophage, NK
   - Placental transfer (1, 3 and 4 but not IgG2), active, from 20 SA
   - Binding to prot G and A of staphelococcus
2. IgA
   - Subclasses: α 1,2
   - Alternate pathway: Aggregate
   - Cellular fixation: Epthelial cells
   - Mucosal immunity
   - Regulation of the bacterial flora: bacteriost in synergy with Lactoferin
3. IgM
   - Cellular fixation: BCR of LB
   - Natural Ac: ABO agglutinin irregular
4. IgD
   - Cellular fixation: BCR of LB
   - increase during pregnancy
5. IgE
   - Alternate pathway: Aggregate
   - Cellular fixation: Mast cells, Macrophage

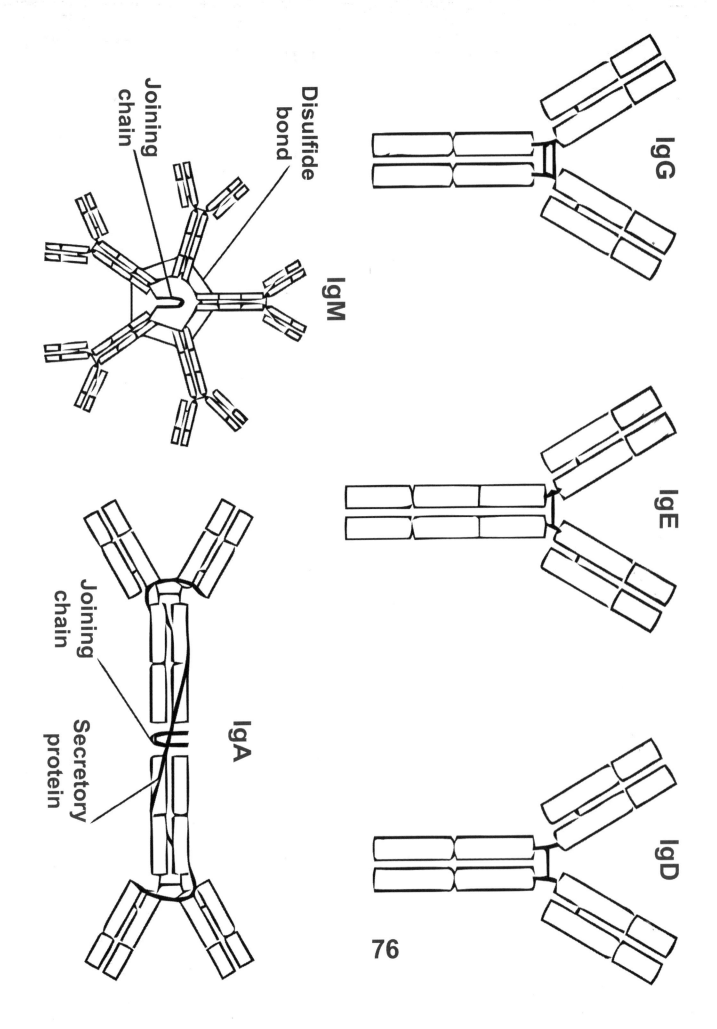

IgG

IgM

Joining
chain

Disulfide
bond

IgE

IgA

Joining
chain

Secretory
protein

IgD

76

HYPERSENSITIVITY I

IgE-dependent phenomenon related to the release of preformed and neoformed mediators by mast cells and basophils in the presence of an allergen.

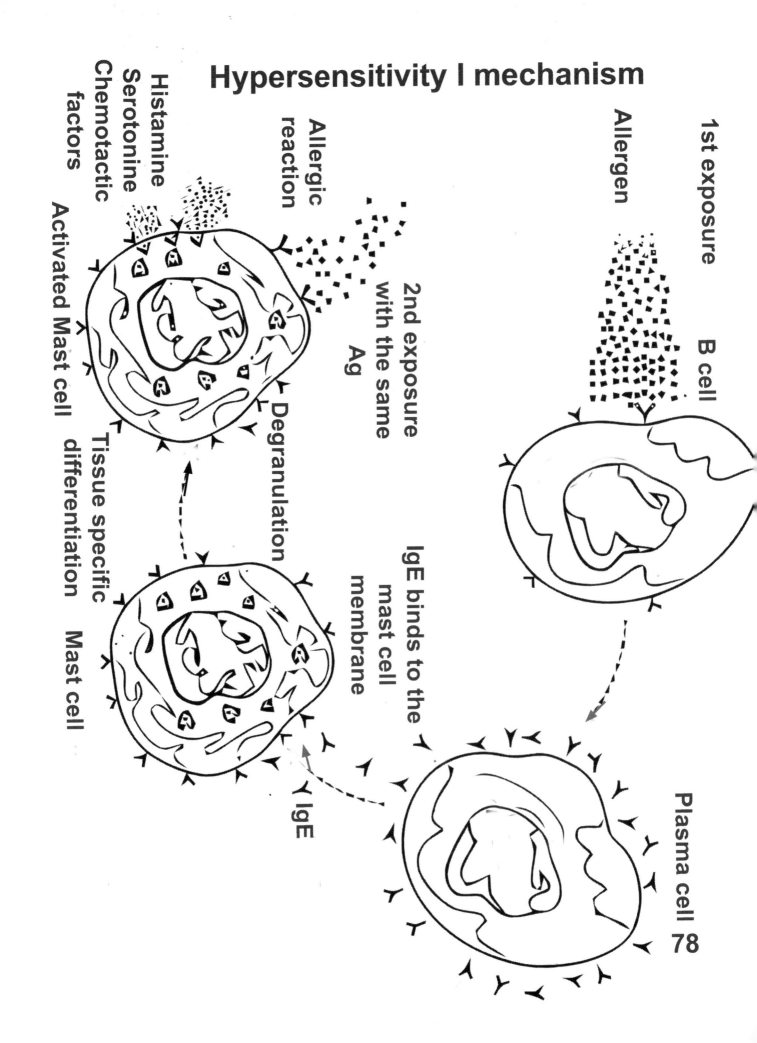

Hypersensitivity I mechanism

PRECIPITATION AND AGGLUTINATION REACTIONS

Definition : formation of a three-dimensional antibody-Ag network, which exists only in the presence of multivalent Ag (multiple epitopes and multivalent antibodies (at least 2 antibody sites > Fab are never precipitating) : Avidity

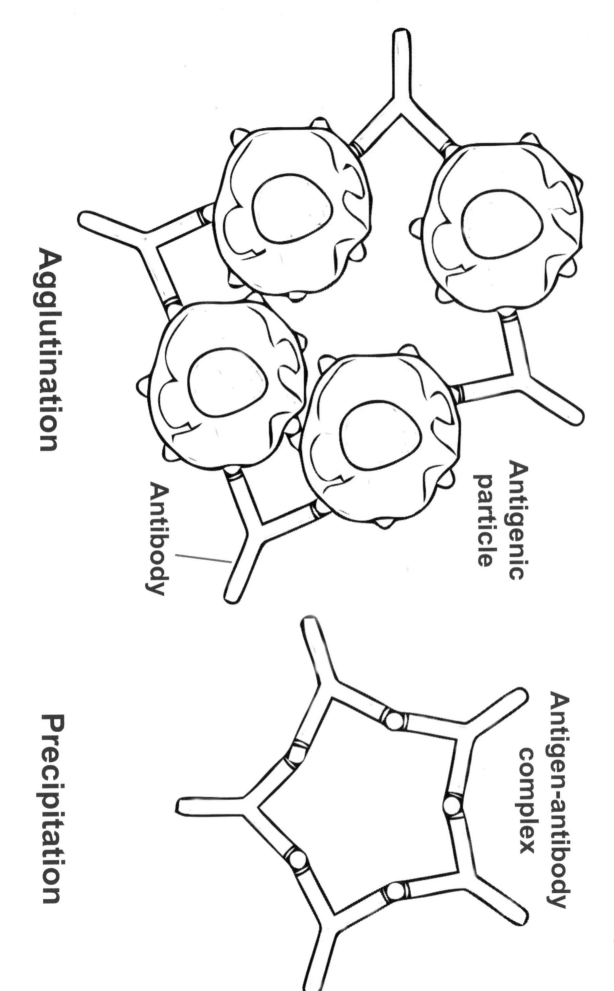

Agglutination

Antibody

Antigenic
particle

Precipitation

Antigen-antibody
complex

80

MONOCLONAL GAMMOPATHIES

Kahler disease (Multiple Myeloma):
Malignant monoclonal proliferation of plasma cells
Lesions often disseminated, rarely localized: plasmacytoma or plasma cell lymphoma
Production of a monoclonal Ig, often complete, exceptionally incomplete
IgG 60% IgA 20% or IgD 1 - 2% (GALDEM)
40%: release of monomers or dimers of identical light chains into the blood and urine = Bence Jones proteins (deposits in the renal tubules: renal complications)

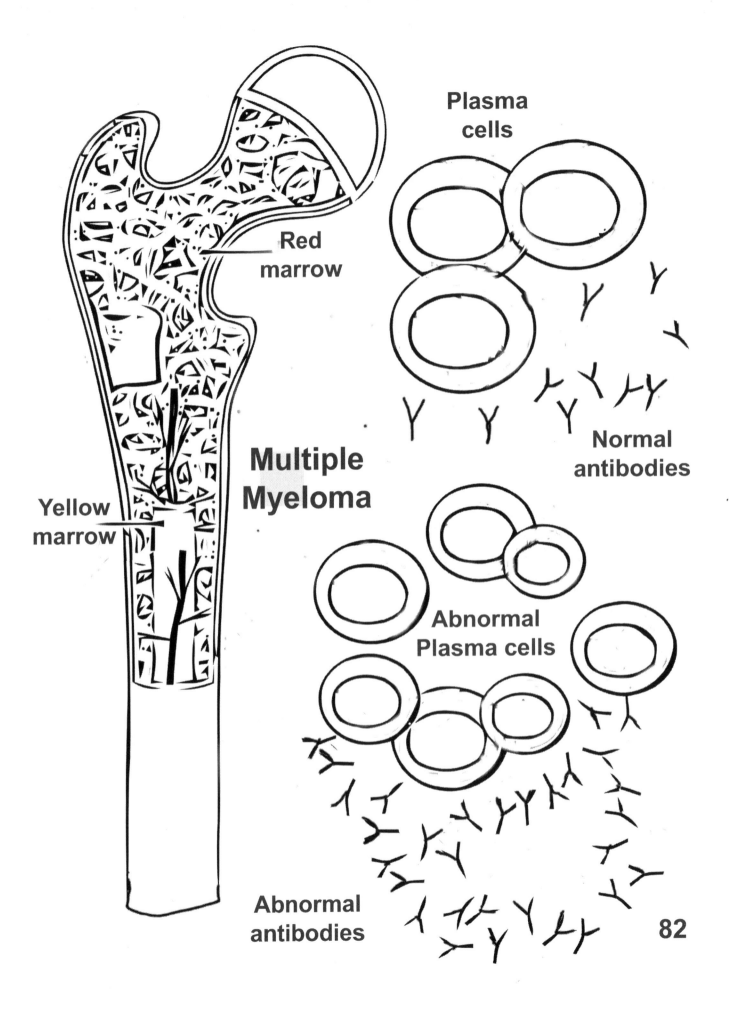

Red marrow

Yellow marrow

Multiple Myeloma

Plasma cells

Normal antibodies

Abnormal Plasma cells

Abnormal antibodies

82

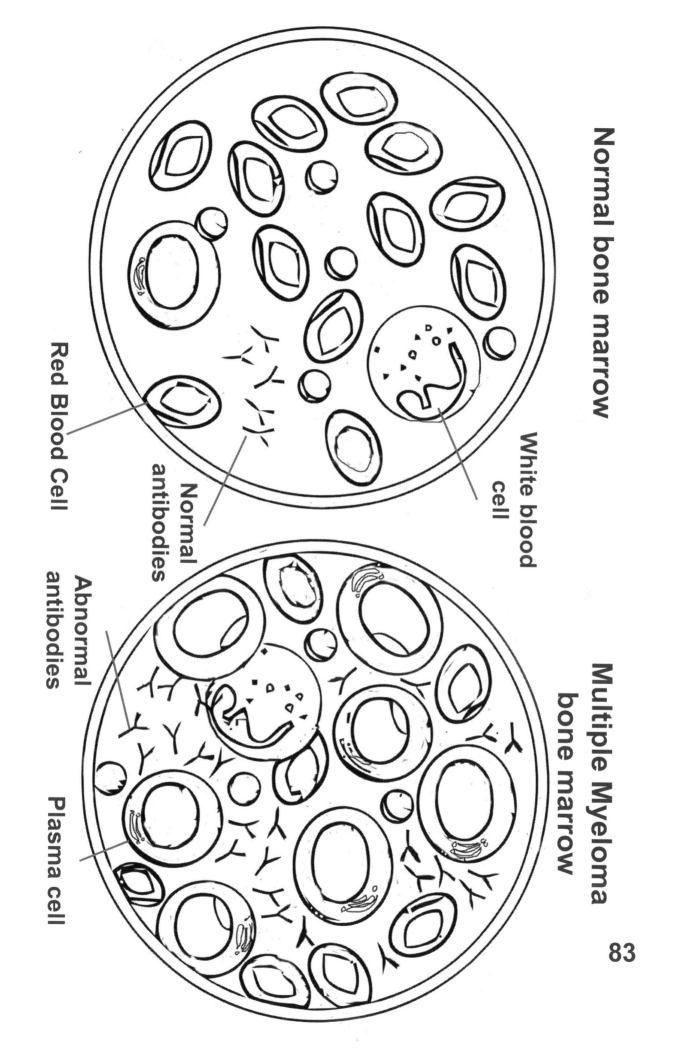

Normal bone marrow

Multiple Myeloma bone marrow

Red Blood Cell

Normal antibodies

White blood cell

Abnormal antibodies

Plasma cell

MONOCLONAL GAMMOPATHIES

LYMPHOMA CLL

Predominantly male disease, subjects over 50 years of age. Tumor infiltration affects bone marrow, lymph nodes, liver, and spleen

Proliferation is monoclonal monomorphic :

LB with low density in IgM, IgD or sometimes IgM+= benign B-CLL with slow progression.

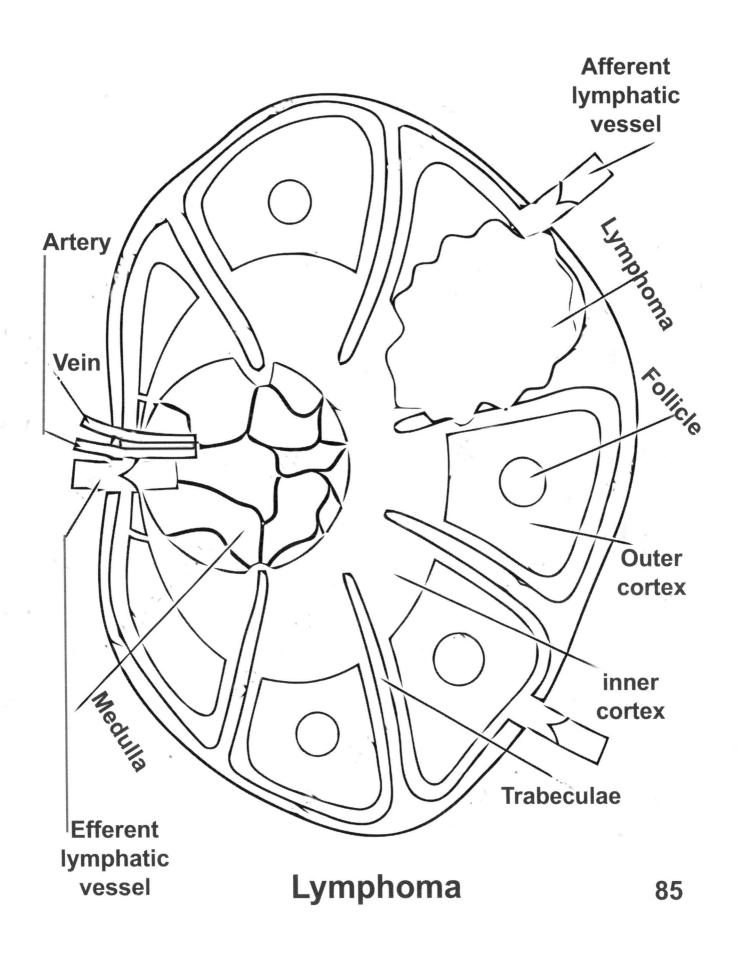

Afferent lymphatic vessel

Lymphoma

Follicle

Artery

Vein

Outer cortex

inner cortex

Medulla

Trabeculae

Efferent lymphatic vessel

Lymphoma

85

ACQUIRED IMMUNODEFICIENCY SYNDROME

Structure of the virus:

HIV is a retrovirus (RNA virus), belonging to the lentivirus family, size 90-120nm. Enveloped virus, the genome contains 9 genes coding for 15 proteins. The most important are :

Env gene: codes for the envelope of the virus

Gag gene: codes for the proteins of the viral capsid "core

Pol genes (Pol25, Pol19): code for enzymes: reverse transcriptase, integrase and protease.

- Envelope :
  - gp 120: allows binding to CD4
  - gp 41: transmembrane protein associated with gp120, necessary for fusion

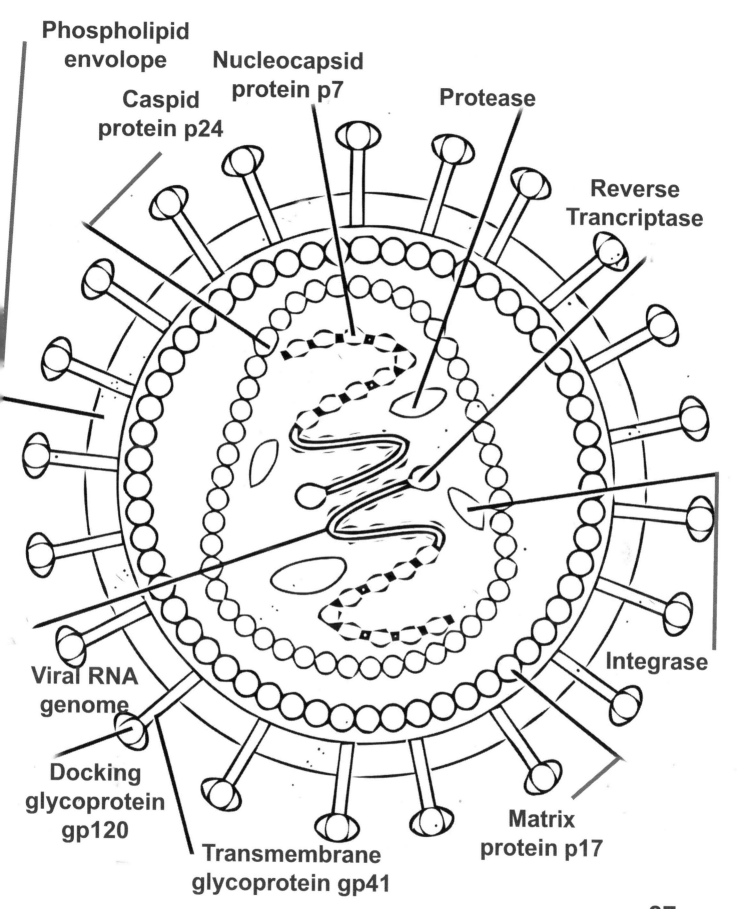

HIV Structure

87

ACQUIRED IMMUNODEFICIENCY SYNDROME

- Virus cycle:
- Binding of gp120 to CD4 of the target cell.
- Conformational change of gp120: unmasks a co-receptor binding site
- Binding of gp120 + co-receptor modifies the structure of the envelope exposure of a hydrophobic region of gp41 hydrophobic region of gp41 = "fusion peptide
- gp41 inserts into the membrane of the target cell, destabilizes it envelope-membrane fusion cell
- Entry of the viral nucleocapsid into the cytoplasm of the target cell
- Decapsidation and release of viral RNA, reverse transcriptase and integrase into the cytoplasm
- Retrotranscription of RNA into DNA, called proviral DNA
- Proviral DNA enters the nucleus, integrates into the cell genome (= Provirus), remains latent
- After activation, the provirus is transcribed into RNAs.
- Translations of viral RNAs into proteins that will be cleaved by viral proteases.
- Proteins + RNA = new virions which will leave the cell by budding of the membrane
- Maturation of virions after budding.

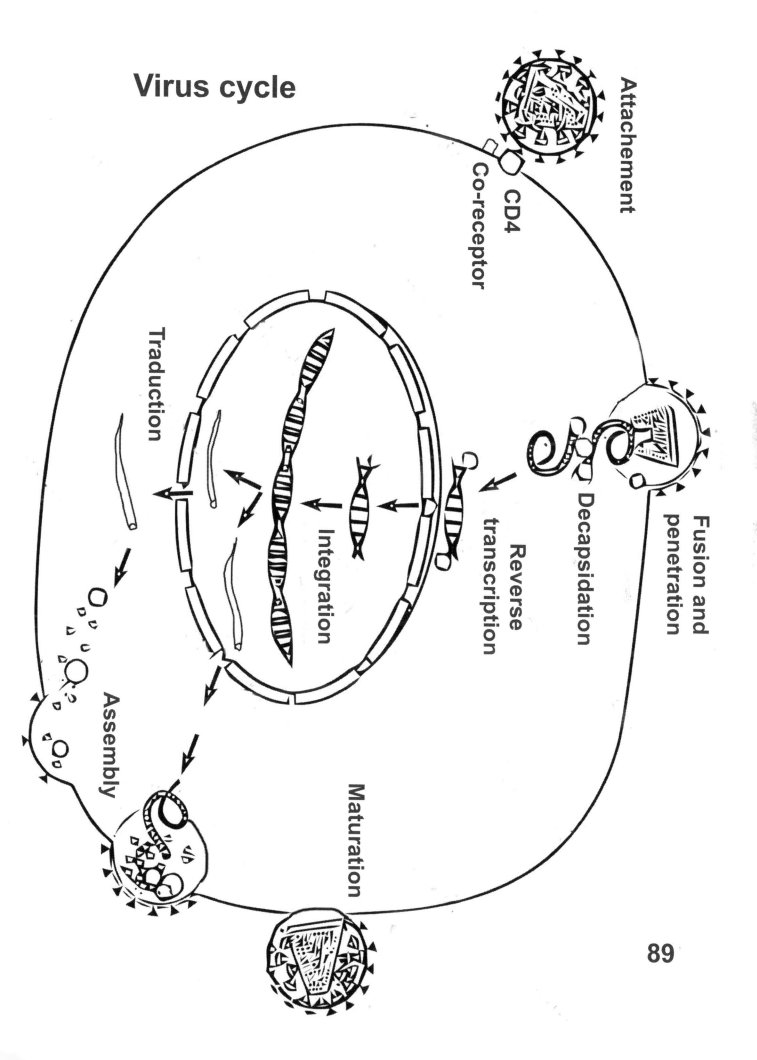

Virus cycle

Attachement

Co-receptor

CD4

Traduction

Integration

Reverse
transcription

Decapsidation

Fusion and
penetration

Assembly

Maturation

89

Printed in Great Britain
by Amazon

85372577R00052